"... an invaluable guide for raising a healthy family ..."

Dr. Earl Mindell
Vitamin Bible and *Vitamin Bible
for Your Kids*

"... [This] book could be the best friend a caring parent can have in the often lonely battle to save their children's health, freedom and, especially, their love, which [Sandy Gooch] wisely grants highest priority.

Even the curious reader, who doesn't care a fig about good food and health, will be rewarded with a treasure house of advice on how to develop an honest, loving relationship with just about anyone."

James J. Julian, M.D.
Medical Director,
Julian Holistic Medical Center

"... practical, common-sense ideas for everyday healthful living ..."

Dale Alexander
Arthritis and Common Sense
and *Good Health and Common
Sense*

"... Sandy's a favorite guest on TV with her helpful hints on health ... this book will enhance her popularity ..."

Dr. Arnold Pike, D.C.
Producer/Host,
Viewpoint on Nutrition TV show

"Sandy Gooch has provided a wonderful information source and guide book for all the mothers and fathers who would like to raise their children on quality, nutritional programs."

Dr. Rob Krakovitz

If You Love Me, Don't Feed Me Junk!

Sandy Gooch

Reston Publishing Company, Inc.
A Prentice Hall Company
Reston, Virginia

Library of Congress Cataloging in Publication Data

Gooch, Sandy.
    If you love me, don't feed me junk!

    1. Food, Natural.   2. Food, Junk.   3. Nutrition.
I. Title.
TX369.G66   1983   613.2   83-10962
ISBN 0-8359-3029-7

Editing and interior design
by Ginger Sasser DeLacey.

© 1983 by
Reston Publishing Company, Inc.
A Prentice-Hall Company
Reston, Virginia

10   9   8   7   6   5   4   3   2   1

Printed in the United States of America

Contents

Contents

Foreword

As one who has long been interested in the positive value of vitamins for you and your children, I can't help but admire Sandy Gooch, who has also fostered the nutrition movement over the years.

To me, Sandy encompasses winning ingredients of good health. In her own way, she possesses "Vitamin E" attributes.

She's—

Enthusiastic—always exuding a spirited flair towards life, always inquisitive, always energized in her quest for truth.

Enlightening—constantly radiating warmth as she shares spiritual insight with her fellow human beings

Educational—never-ending in her desire to spread information and knowledge about health and nutrition (surely all this stemmed from her many years as a schoolteacher)

Empathetic—from her childhood days she has always sensed the needs and feelings of others and has selflessly given of her time and energy to enrich people's lives

Entertaining—she knows how to tell her story in a charming, charismatic fashion, projecting a style all her own

You'll find all these special Vitamin E's throughout the pages of her book. I'm happy she's making this contribution which I feel is an invaluable guide for raising a healthy family.

Earl Mindell, R.Ph., Ph.D.

Author of *Vitamin Bible* and
Vitamin Bible for Your Kids

Foreword

I have been looking for just such a work to enable my patients to move over to the healthy way. They sit in my office and nod their heads as if they knew exactly how to do it culinarily and emotionally.

There are a number of books out now with recipes omitting sugar, salt, fat and white flour. But my patients, usually mothers, are intimidated by their children, their spouses, and their in-laws. Those people are addicted to the stuff.

Gradualism seems to be the way to go, along with educational insights. I am trying to get the schools to understand that someone is going to hit them with a law suit for tooth decay if they don't get the candy machines out of their halls. You are right, the children are often the best ones to teach their own parents.

You have contributed a great work for the millions out there struggling to change just a few things in their environment. You have covered just about every contingency that might come up when the converted cook in the family is hit with the invidious attacks of the sugar addicts.

Keep at it.

Lendon H. Smith, M.D.

Physician and Surgeon

Foreword

My concern for health and healthful food consumption has been documented many times over. There is no way that I could, in good conscience, endorse a product or program without being totally and completely convinced of its integrity and of the personal and professional integrity of the individual promoting it.

Mrs. Gooch and I first met in 1981 at a Health Food Convention in Las Vegas. She was being buttonholed by a food manufacturer who was lamenting the fact that he had lost $10 million in sales because she had failed to accept his product for distribution in her chain of markets.

I admire Mrs. Gooch who has made it, from a business sense, in a field dominated by men and who has also been unrelenting in her decision that only foods that are healthful and nutritious can be distributed in her chain. She does not accept the word of the manufacturer as to the nutritional content of a food item but subjects each item in her store to rigorous laboratory testing.

It has been documented that sugar and white flour are the number one causes of criminal behavior and that table salt is the second highest cause of cancer.

I am aware that eating habits cannot be changed overnight. Mrs. Gooch's diet recommendations are transitional in nature. Even though meat is included in her markets it does not contain additives, chemicals or hormones.

As Americans, we need to look at some sad statistics regarding persons under age thirty-one and the top five causes of mortality: #1 Auto Accidents, #2 Homicides, #3 Suicide, #4 Cancer, #5 Drugs. All of these are too often related to items ingested into the body. It's a cliche, but it's true: We Are What We Eat. It would be well to remember that strong national might is not to be found in weapons and defense, but in strong and healthy minds and bodies.

It is therefore, both inspiring and gratifying to add my strong endorsement of Sandy Gooch's book, *If You Love Me, Don't Feed Me Junk.*

Dick Gregory

Actor/Activist

Acknowledgments

So many people have given so generously of their time and energy and knowledge and love to help make this book come true! To fully describe each person's unique role would take another manuscript almost the length of this one—and I don't think Barbara Lovenvirth, my editor at Reston, would smile on that.

So, all you wonderful people: Dr. Marc Harmon D.D.S., Joyce Virtue Ph.D., Dr. George Meduski MD-Ph.D., Doug Kaufmann, Geoffrey Cheung Ph.D., Alfred J. Plechner D.V.M., Dominick Bosco, Nancy Uyemura, Sue Epstein, Kristin Gooch, Doug Stone, Richard Holmes, Nancy Kelly, Irwin Zucker, Jim and Rosalie Heacock, Sue Baumeister, Julie Aihara, Diana Temple, Terry King, Harry Lederman, Steven Lederman, Don Delong, Anthony Nex, Sharon Louden, Dr. Rob Krakovitz MD, Natasha Trenev, and Rondi and Rich Prescott—

Thank you very much!

I Learned the Hard Way
(My Story)

You're never too young—or too old—to learn to say, "If you love me, don't feed me junk!"

I hope the lesson for you has been—and continues to be—an easy one. I had to learn the hard way. My life had to be threatened for me to begin to understand the importance of a natural foods diet.

Before 1974, I was one of those people who didn't know that nutrition could make a difference in the quality of life. I was a former schoolteacher turned wife and mother who had always been in pretty good physical health. The only allergy I was aware of was one to peanut products. Like millions of other homemakers, I shopped at supermarkets and used convenience foods—and hardly ever gave it a second thought.

Then a bout with the sniffles almost ended my life.

Normally, I didn't go to the doctor just because of the sniffles, but this particular case was persistent, so I made an appointment. My doctor prescribed tetracycline, a common antibiotic. I left her office believing I would feel better soon.

On the contrary. A few days later, I felt so bad I thought I was going to die! I suddenly started shaking uncontrollably. My chest hurt so badly I thought I was having a heart attack. My head wouldn't stop spinning, and if I tried to read, the words on the page just wouldn't stand still!

I had never been so scared in my entire life!

I was rushed to UCLA hospital, but the doctors could not find any cause for the terrible symptoms I was having. Then, as mysteriously as they came on, the symptoms vanished. I left the hospital and tried to forget my sudden, unexplained attack.

1

Two weeks later, I went to the doctor again—this time with an eye infection. Again, she gave me tetracycline. Within minutes, I was in the throes of another, even more violent, attack. My body felt like it was under siege. This time, the symptoms didn't subside in a few hours. My head kept on spinning. My muscles shook uncontrollably. My chest tightened painfully, and I had to struggle with all my might for every breath of air.

I was driven over 100 miles to the Scripps Institute in La Jolla. There, I was examined by scores of experts: allergists, internal medicine specialists, and medical researchers. I was given every kind of test imaginable, but everyone was totally baffled. Not one doctor had the slightest idea what was causing my horrible attacks—or what to do to stop them.

After three days, the symptoms subsided all by themselves. I stayed on at Scripps, and the tests continued, in vain.

On the evening of my fifth day there, I took a sip of diet soda. Suddenly, my body started tingling from head to toe. Within minutes, I was in agony all over again. I felt like I was going to die! As a matter of fact, I almost did die. This attack cut off my air supply. No matter how hard I tried, I just couldn't force my lungs to breathe!

A nurse realized that my life was in immediate danger and gave me a shot of benadryl, a powerful antihistamine. The attack subsided. I still felt very ill, but at least I could breathe.

Still, no one could tell me what was happening to me, why it was happening, and when it might happen again. After a total of ten days at Scripps, I left—no closer to having any answers than I'd been at the moment of my first attack.

The only thing I had come closer to was death. When I went to bed each night, I honestly didn't know if I would wake up the next morning.

I started going to doctor after doctor, searching for the answers that would help me regain my health, for I surely had lost it. Why, I could hardly carry out my day-to-day activities! I never knew when I might again be reduced to a suffocating, dizzy, pain-wracked invalid. No doctor could help me.

One doctor even expressed his frustration by pronouncing, "It's all in your head." As if my brush with death at the Scripps Institute had been a figment of my imagination! And the imaginations of the hospital staff that saved my life!

Nevertheless, this doctor suggested that my problem might be psychosomatic. He said I should go home and examine my life, so I went home and sat under a pine tree and thought about my life.

I was in despair. Never had I felt more alone. Nobody understood what I was going through. Nobody had the answer. Nobody even knew if there ever *would* be an answer! And now they were even starting to suggest that I was really suffering from a mental problem and that my dire physical distress was all caused by my mind!

What made me feel even worse was that *I was close to believing it myself!* What else could be the answer? Maybe I was mentally ill!

Yet, somewhere deep down inside me, a small voice kept telling me that it wasn't in my mind and that I really could be healthy again ... somehow.

I was saved by my father. My dad played the leading role in my struggle to regain health. Ever since my close call at Scripps, he had been applying his skills and knowledge as a research biologist to my problem. Dad believed in me. He knew me so well that he was certain there had to be a physical reason for what was happening to me. My father did not accept the words of the doctors who were dismissing my illness as psychosomatic. Dad said, "I know her. I've lived with her and observed her. That's simply not the case—what's wrong with her is not psychosomatic."

Dad went to work finding the real answers. He ferreted out bits of information piece by piece. He read books and articles. He called up people and asked questions. He wrote letters. My father worked long, hard hours because he felt he still had a responsibility towards me, his child, to do all he could to improve my health.

Finally, where the doctors had failed, Dad succeeded. My father found the answers.

My original attacks, he explained, were allergic reactions to the antibiotic, tetracycline. My first reaction took many days to begin because I wasn't fully sensitized to the antibiotic—my body wasn't primed to react against the intruder. My first dose primed me. As subsequent doses entered my system, my reaction grew in strength and violence.

Then, when I was treated with the drug a second time, not only was the reaction brought on sooner, but it was even more violent.

As for the attack at Scripps, Dad reasoned that something in the diet soda was the cause. He investigated the ingredients and found the culprit: bromelated vegetable oil. It sounds harmless, but it almost killed me. This additive has the power to inhibit the body's antihistamine, which protects us against severe reactions to allergens, toxins, and infections.

My body's supply of antihistamine was already severely depleted from fighting off the original assault by the antibiotic. The bromelated vegetable oil (also known as bromelate acetate) instantly inactivated what little antihistamine I had left in my body. I was left almost totally vulnerable to the allergic attack of the tetracycline that was still seeping out of my liver and kidneys into my bloodstream.

Thanks to my father, I took my first step towards health. I realized that there was a definite, physical cause for my illness.

Nevertheless, there were many more steps to take before I fully regained my health. Although I was home from the hospital, I still felt horrible. In fact, I was so sick that Kristin, my daughter, was placed in a foster home. Friends came to take care of me while my husband was at work. (One of these friends was Nancy Uyemura, the artist and teacher who illustrated this book.)

I knew I had to avoid tetracycline and diet soda, but I suspected it wasn't going to be that simple. I tried my best to *act* healthy. After a brief convalescence, I slowly resumed my household responsibilities and slowly started to feel better. I went to work on the very first meal I would prepare myself since coming home from the hospital: roast chicken.

Imagine how proud I was when I served that chicken! I thought I was on the road to becoming my old healthy self again!

Then, I ate half a drumstick, and nearly found myself back in the hospital! Within five minutes of my first bite, I felt the dizziness and the chest pains and the tightness of breath coming over me. I started pacing the kitchen floor, wringing my hands ... and crying.

I was utterly devastated! This attack dealt an even heavier blow to my hopes for recovery than the nearly fatal one at Scripps! After all, I hadn't been near a doctor, drugs, or diet soda for weeks!

Or so I thought. Dad—whose research into my problem never stopped—found out that much of the chicken that comes into California from out-of-state is actually *dipped* in tetracycline!

That fact not only made me sick but very angry as well. I was angry when I found out that I had, in total ignorance, eaten something mortally dangerous to me. It seemed criminally negligent to allow food to be contaminated with potentially hazardous chemicals and to hide that fact from consumers.

For weeks and weeks after the chicken episode, I felt like a human guinea pig. Some foods made me sick; others didn't. I didn't know what to expect when I took a bite of food! There was no way to be really sure. Many foods that I thought were pure, because I had once eaten them with no reaction, would surprise me with mini-attacks—evidence of some form of contamination by a harmful additive.

And the more my father investigated our food supply, the more evidence he found of contamination with harmful chemicals. Even though Dad had never had more than a passing interest in so-called "health foods," the conclusion he reached was firm and clear: *The additives in processed food could and would continue to make me ill for the rest of my life. If I wanted to be healthy, I had to put myself on a totally natural foods diet.*

What did a "natural foods diet" mean?

It meant this: *No refined flour or sugar. No artificial additives. No artificial flavors, colors, or preservatives. No caffeine. No hydrogenated vegetable oil.*

What was most remarkable was that Dad himself had never been on any kind of natural foods diet. He wasn't coming from the position, "I've done it and it's been good for me." He reached his conclusion through his own research into my problem.

In fact, Dad's personal and professional life couldn't have been further from a pro "natural foods" position. My father was, in essence, part of the medical business. He owned his own pharmaceutical house and formulated drugs for doctors, dentists, and veterinarians. He had always included lots of soda, coffee, ice cream, meat, fat, and sugar in his diet.

Amazingly, Dad performed a perfect 180-degree turnaround. He not only told me to start on a natural foods diet, but he also learned how (and then taught me how) to obtain and prepare a lot of these new foods!

So with Dad's constant supervision, I put myself on a totally natural foods diet. I got better. Slowly.

It was three months before I even felt there was a chance for me to live a full, healthy life. It was nine months before I knew I was really on my way towards achieving that goal.

There were plateaus—times when I felt "Wow! This must be it! I'm as healthy as I can be!" Then a few months later, I would look back and realize that I had still been getting better. I was constantly taking small steps forward.

After a year, I finally felt healed. Even then, there were setbacks. Once, I slipped and had two glasses of beer at a picnic. Suddenly, I was whisked all the way back to the beginning! I felt like I was going to die! The chest pain radiated down to my arms. I was dizzy and disoriented. I was in agony for three weeks.

My father calmly approached it from a strictly scientific basis. Cause and effect. It had to be additives in the beer.

I felt angry again, because I didn't know there were any additives in beer. Once again, there was no warning on the label.

That's when I really started thinking about our food supply. I read a lot of books and talked to a lot of people. I learned that I was not alone, that millions of people were also suffering from ill health because of the impurities in their food, air, and water.

Actually, I came to feel that I was one of the lucky ones. My reactions were so violent that I simply had to find the answer—or die. There are millions of people, I learned, whose reactions are not violent enough to threaten their lives—just severe enough to chip away at their health a little at a time and to gradually rob them of life's energy, vibrancy, and excitement. These millions may never find the answers. They may never be driven to find optimum health because they may never realize that they are not as healthy as they could be.

I thought there were many people who might benefit from my experience. I knew there were many who could be helped if they had access to the same wholesome food that I found could maintain my health, so I started Mrs. Gooch's, a natural foods supermarket. My standards for stocking the shelves were—and continue to be—straightforward, based on my father's research. *No artificial additives of any kind. No artificial colors, flavors, or preservatives. No white flour. No refined sugar. No caffeine. No hydrogenated vegetable oil.*

In the same way my father helped me keep an eye on my diet, my entire staff keeps a diligent eye on every product that comes into the store to make sure this philosophy of natural food is never compromised. The concept was embraced by so many people that now there are several Mrs. Gooch's markets.

My life was truly transformed—as well as saved—by my father's love. When I say it's never too late—or too early—for a parent's loving, determined concern for a child's well-being to benefit the child, I am speaking from experience.

Dad, thank you. This book is dedicated to your memory.

Cover art and chapter opening illustrations
by Nancy Uyemura.

Kids Eat the Darnedest Things drawings and recipes
by the children of my 1969-1970 kindergarten class.

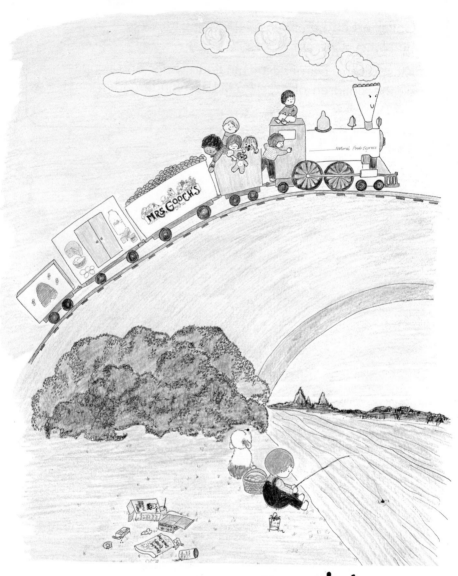

you can do it!

1

Our children come into the world crying, "Love me! Feed me!"

We do love them, so we feed them the best food we can. And something wonderful happens. They grow.

They learn to say, "Momma ... Poppa ... doggie!"

But then something crazy happens. They learn to say "No!"

"No, I don't want vegetables!"

"No, I don't want oatmeal!"

"I want Choco-sweets!"

"Give me a candybar!"

Why on earth does this happen?

Maybe the sweet little brats on TV have hypnotized our children?

Maybe every other child in town is hooked on Choco-sweets?

Maybe while babysitting, Grandma and Grandpa ignorantly initiated the children into the perverse, perditious pleasures of Choco-sweets and candybars?

Maybe Dad is secretly a junk food junkie?

Worst of all, maybe somewhere, sometime, somehow, we had something to do with teaching our children to say, "If you love me, feed me Choco-sweets!"

"Feed me Greaseburgers!"

"Feed me candybars!"

"Feed me Fatty-fries!"

"Feed me Purple Chemi-Doo-Dads!"

We want to just cry out: "I love you! Why don't you want your raw vegetables and wheat germ? They're good for you!"

Where, we wonder, did our children learn to be so very suspicious of the food we believe is good for them? So suspicious that every child psychologist and pediatrician seems to warn, "Never tell a child that something you want him to eat is good for him."

What a terrible thing for a parent to feel defensive about!

When our children are less than enthusiastic about the good food we want to give them and the skills we want to teach them, it frustrates our love for them—as well as our nutritional goals.

That's why this book is about food *and* love.

I believe we can express our love for our children, provide them with the best food, and teach them the ways of healthy eating. I don't believe for a minute that we need to act defensive about it, either. If we know *how* to tell our children what food is good for them, we can do it without acting the least bit shy about it. They'll get the message, too.

As an owner of the natural foods markets that bear my name, I talk to thousands of parents who are trying to provide the best nutrition for their children. Their stories are success stories—otherwise, I couldn't write this book.

But I also hear about their problems. I hear about the obstacles and challenges these parents come up against, and eventually overcome. I hear about the Choco-sweets for breakfast and the Purple Chemi-Doo-Dads under the bed. I hear about the nutritious home-made lunches traded for Greaseburgers, Fatty-fries, and cola. I hear about the neighbors, in-laws, school cafeterias, and friends who bombard children with junk—and the TV commercials that demoniacally convince children and parents alike that junk food is "part of a balanced diet."

But I also hear about the children who learn to reject unhealthy food both at home and away. I hear about the children who even turn on their friends to the joys and benefits of healthy eating.

I talk to a lot of children, too. And I find them a lot more receptive to finding out "what's good for them" than the experts lead us to believe.

So I want to assure you that, following the suggestions in this book, you *will* make progress in guiding your children to a healthier way of eating. Using these strategies, you will be able to teach your children about food and help them build habits of healthy eating that can last a lifetime.

I know that all of us parents sometimes wonder if our efforts are worthwhile. Just the other day, Sarah—one mother whose progress in improving her family's diet I have followed and marvelled at for years— shrugged her shoulders and said to me, "Sandy, I just don't know if it's worth all the trouble!"

Sarah seemed really concerned, so I asked her if any of her children were ill. She said they were all fine.

I asked her if her teenagers were doing well in school. She said they made the honor roll again, but her son's involvement with designing and building model airplanes and her daughter's editorship of the school paper were competing with sports for their after-school time.

I asked Sarah if she had reason to believe her children were unhappy or in some kind of trouble. Sarah said, "No."

Finally, a bit exasperated, I said, "Sarah, dear, what is the problem?"

"They told me they just don't like whole wheat pizza, and they want to go out for a 'real' pizza every now and then."

"Sarah," I said, with a comforting smile, "how far you've really come!"

We looked into each other's faces for a few moments, and then both burst into laughter at the same time.

We all have moments when we feel like Sarah—times when the slightest setback can make us temporarily forget all the progress we've really made.

I'm going to tell you the same thing I told Sarah, and what I tell others who confess their doubts about how much they've actually accomplished: Your efforts will not be in vain. Guiding your children into a healthy, natural foods diet is one of the greatest ways you can show your love. You will be boosting their opportunities to have a healthy, productive, happy life.

This book is about more than how to get your children to eat good food. The text, projects, and recipes are designed to help you overcome the *human* problems you will encounter, but you will find no elaborate system of punishments and rewards. My approach relies on building your children's self-esteem and confidence.

I believe the best way to teach anybody anything is through communication, practice, and aggressive faith in their ability to learn. So that's what you'll find in this book.

Please don't worry about whether your children are too old or too young. Children of all ages are extemely receptive to this kind of information when it's presented to them in a form they can understand. I know this from my many experiences in which children have responded to natural foods and to information about natural foods.

Young schoolchildren walk right by the Mrs. Gooch's market in Hermosa Beach, California, on their way to and from school each day. We happen to have our natural foods demonstration booth set up in the front window. When the store first opened, the children were a little suspicious. They would ask what kind of food we were preparing—and then move on. Sometimes they'd say "Yecch! Who needs natural foods!"

But then they ventured into the store far enough to sample a taste. And then another. And then another. Before long, our demonstration booth was a regular stop on the way home from school. I know there had to be several children who walked many blocks out of their way to sample the natural goodies. I also know that quite a few parents came into the market for the first time at their children's urging—because of the good food they found there.

And every time I lead a group of schoolchildren on a classroom tour through one of my markets, I am approached by new faces the very next day:

"My daughter said we have to stop eating sugar and processed food!"

"My kids refuse to eat their Choco-sweets anymore! What miracle did you perform?"

"My son insisted that I come in here and buy some natural food!"

These were parents of fourth graders. But first graders and teenagers respond the same way. They are all receptive. They all want to be as healthy as they can.

Our children never really stop saying, "If you love me, don't feed me junk!"

We just need to learn how to hear that message and answer it.

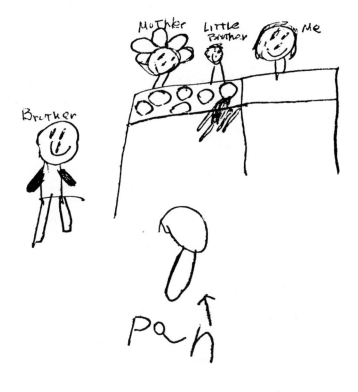

Sausages

Buy a box of sausages and go home. Get some eggs and fry them in a little bit of black oil.

Put the eggs on a plate. Fry the sausages in a pan and serve these with the eggs.

Whoever wants any can eat it. Whoever doesn't has to make something else.

Debbie Castellon

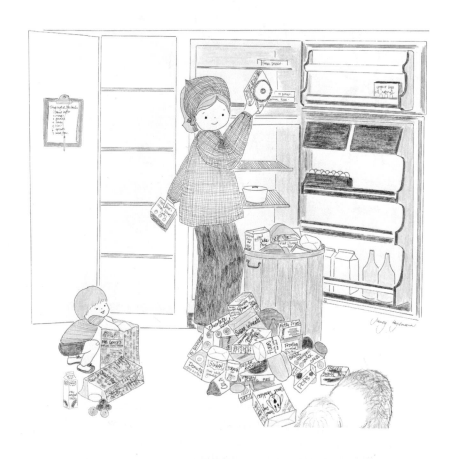

Start With Yourself

2

A mother tells me she is convinced a natural foods diet is best for her children. Then she asks, "Sandy, where do I start?"

I'm ready with an answer:

"Start with yourself."

Once I met, and had over for dinner, Sheila, a charming twenty-eight year old woman, and Johnny, her three year old son. Sheila suffers from hypoglycemia and is very overweight. She told me that when she was in high school she had temper tantrums and flew into rages with the least provocation. Everybody in her family had the same problem. Nobody tried to find out the cause or correct the condition. They just dismissed it by saying, "It runs in the family."

When Sheila was pregnant, she was nauseated for the entire nine months. She had no energy, no pep, and was absolutely miserable.

Finally, Sheila discovered that she was hypoglycemic. She talked to a nutritionist, who advised her to switch to natural foods and take some vitamin supplements.

Sheila appeared very sincere and enthusiastic about changing her diet—and her son's diet. "I don't want Johnny to go through what I went through," she said, "so I'm changing the whole family's diet."

And yet, when she started talking about Johnny, she said he "didn't have that much sugar anymore." She went on to say that he loved lollipops and popsicles, so she was keeping some of those items in the house. She explained she was doing it "for my son," and "it isn't that much."

I asked Sheila if *she* took advantage of having the candy in the house. She said *every* now and then she did.

I don't tell this story to point a finger at someone who's failing. Eventually, as she learned more about food and about her own problem, Sheila realized that what was "not that much" could sometimes be too much.

Sheila eventually realized that you can't go halfway with yourself. If you want your children to have a deep, growing commitment to health and a good diet, you must start with your own deep, growing commitment. Keep your end of the bargain.

Your child is going to learn from your example. His commitment will keep pace with yours. If you go halfway, so will he. Children, after all, don't do what we say. They do what we do.

How can you tell a child sugar is bad for him when you're flying into a coffee-and-doughnut-induced low blood sugar rage?

If you keep something in the house that is not nutritious, are you keeping your end of the bargain? The very real presence of doughnuts, soda pop, candybars, and frozen plastic pies is stimulation to your child. As long as they're around, the message is "This is OK."

Be ruthlessly honest. If you're keeping junk around the house for yourself, don't blame your child. Don't say "The child can't do without it," when it's *you* who can't.

Your child *can* do without it—unless you convince him otherwise. If you say, "Eat this whole wheat bread because it's good for you," but then say, "I keep a few Purple Chemi-Doo-Dads around the house because you can't do without them," guess which lesson your child learns?

He learns that he can't do without Purple Chemi-Doo-Dads.

If you want your natural foods revolution to be successful—if you want your child to learn to make nutritional decisions that will lead to a healthy life—*you* must make the decisions first.

What Are Your Goals?

At the beginning of every school year, I made a written statement of my goals. I asked myself: "What do I want my students to know and be able to do by the end of the year?"

I had academic goals, social goals, and emotional goals. I wanted them to reach certain levels of proficiency in reading, writing, and arithmetic, but I also wanted them to be better at getting along with one another.

Why don't you make a list of your goals?

Here, too, start with yourself. What are your goals for yourself? You can be as broad or as narrow in scope as you wish. For example, you might list as your first goal, "to have a happy, healthy life." Or you might write, "to be able to get through the day with plenty of energy to spare."

What are your goals for your child?

It's not my role to prescribe goals for you. However, I am writing this book with certain goals in mind, goals that I believe are worthy. I believe you should know, up front, what I believe is important.

In my former role as a schoolteacher, I saw several books and teacher's manuals telling parents how to make sure their children could read, write, and do arithmetic before they got to the first grade. As important as these skills are, I have always felt that if we want our children to stay inquisitive, curious, and perceptive—which is how they are when they come into the world—we need to do much, much more than teach numbers and letters. Numbers and letters are only tools.

There are other important lessons to teach children. I believe a sense of responsibility for their own health and growth—and responsibility for the health and growth of the planet—are important lessons. In today's mechanized world, it's easy to forget our reliance on—and responsibility to—the natural world. Every day, we are learning more about the disastrous consequences of our forgetting this responsibility. We are also becoming reacquainted with the many benefits we can enjoy when we harmonize with nature.

I believe that over-processed, mass-produced, devitalized foods containing artificial ingredients are manifestations of that dangerous lapse of memory and respect. Learning about natural foods can help reawaken in our children a fascination and respect for all that is living. Everything that is truly food comes from living matter—not from a chemist's test tube. It is my goal that our children will not only learn the relationship between food and life, but that they will express that harmony throughout their lives.

In learning about food, a child can learn a lot more than nutrition. He can learn about science as he observes the many relationships among people, animals, plants, food elements, and chemicals.

Many of the activities in this book involve cooking. Cooking skills are excellent preparation for science and math. Not only do you learn how to follow an experimental plan (recipe) and how to manipulate tools and ingredients for a desired effect—but you also learn to methodically observe the results ... so you can do better the next time.

Learning about food can stimulate a child's social and emotional development. As a classroom teacher, I could not get away from the fact that I needed to have the children's social and emotional goals in mind right along with the academic ones. It was undeniable that the children were vulnerable to these lessons in the classroom.

The same is true in this book. Social and emotional development will take place as you teach your child about food. As this book progresses, you'll hear me talk about self-image, confidence, independence, and communication. After all, food is a lot more than physical nourishment, so learning about food must be a lot more than learning about nutrition.

For example, one of the things we need to know about ourselves is that our efforts can produce desirable results: We can be effective. We can have goals, act on them, and achieve them. Learning to cook—to produce a meal that satisfies hunger, nourishes, and provides an occasion for a happy gathering of loved ones—is one of the most fundamental and effective ways of giving a child (or any person) that very important feeling of confidence.

Lifelong Lessons Are Best

Remember how you felt back in school when you were required to learn something by rote? Do you remember any of those lessons?

Although rote learning can be effective for some very simple mechanical skills, my goal in teaching my own child about nutrition has been more ambitious. I have always wanted Kristin to internalize these lessons so that she will be able to make her own choices when I'm not around to help her. Naturally, no parent can always stand over a child and tell her what's right or wrong. When a parent tries to do that, the child isn't really learning anything but devotion to authority.

I want Kristin to be able to figure things out *by* and *for* herself. In later years, this pride in herself will show in the kind of person she becomes, the career she chooses, the perseverance she relies on in going after her own goals. It will show in what she does for herself and for those around her.*

Whatever "it" is you're trying to teach your child, you know she's really got "it" when she freely makes the choice. If your child chooses certain foods only when you're around to police her, she hasn't got "it." But if she makes the choices you have tried to teach her even when she's by herself or with her friends, then you know you've accomplished something wonderful.

I was really delighted recently with Kristin's response to the opportunity to choose freely. She and a group of her friends were planning a weekend trip to Lake Arrowhead, a recreational area two hours northeast of Los Angeles. There are plenty of fast food restaurants up there, but Kristin asked me to supply the groceries for the trip.

I told her to make a list, and I was very curious to see what she would write. Without giving it a whole lot of thought, Kristin wrote down: tuna, trail mix, lettuce, whole wheat bread, fresh fruit, natural snacks ... . Then she passed the list over and said, "And anything you can think of that would be good."

I was really delighted. You see, I have never forced Kristin into any particular pattern of eating. She always makes her own choices. Kristin knows I *expect* her to make her own choices.

Your child can understand what you expect of her—and what you expect of yourself—if you tell her your goals and how you plan to go about achieving them.

---

*Another benefit of starting early is that if your child ever strays, it will be that much easier for her to find her way back. Tricia Dix, Director of Nutrition at Mrs. Gooch's, grew up in a "natural foods home." Tricia's mother read Adelle Davis' books and learned all about the value of good natural foods and food supplements. Tricia still remembers receiving her vitamins in an egg cup every morning. Nevertheless, in college Tricia did stray from the healthy eating patterns her mother set down for her. But then something happened that brought her back. A close friend of Tricia's suffered from a case of lupus that the conventional doctors could not help. A wholistic doctor put Tricia's friend on a totally natural foods diet, with supplementation, and, three years later, there were no signs of the disease. Her friend's consistent devotion to her natural foods diet reawakened in Tricia the memory of her mother's dedication and love. Her friend's success made such an impact on Tricia that she decided to devote her life to promoting health through a natural foods lifestyle.

Define Your Terms

Make a list of the terms that you feel need to be defined. Some of the words on my personal list are: natural food, regular food, junk food, processed food, convenience food, organic food, nutritious food, and health food.

Language is one of the most powerful tools we have—and one of the most necessary. When we have a name for something, we have power that we didn't have before. It you think about it for a minute, you'll begin to understand how confusing it could be if people didn't agree on what names to use for one another, for places, and for things. Now, imagine what a barrier to understanding it could be if your child didn't have a clear idea of what you meant when you said, "natural food," or "junk food," or "nutritious."

Defining terms always involves value judgments. For example, you can make a reasonable attempt to define "natural food" by using scientific statements. You can say, as I do, that natural food is any food that has no artificial colors, flavors, or preservatives, and that contains no white flour, no refined sugar, no caffeine, and no hydrogenated vegtable oil. No food that has been drastically altered from its original nutritional state by refining and processing can be called natural.

I hope this definition works as well for you as it does for me. Nevertheless, you will run into people whose values allow them to use a quite different definition—a definition that allows them to call white sugar "natural!"

Some of my friends in the natural foods business spent several days in Federal Trade Commission hearings trying to come up with an acceptable definition of the word "natural." Part of the problem was that across the aisle were attorneys from the processed food industry who questioned every area of the definition that required the least bit of value judgment. They argued that white sugar was "natural" because nothing "artificial" was added to it.

It was, of course, contrary to the interests of the processed food industry to have the government establish real standards for what could be called natural. Some attorneys for the processed food industry actually wanted the word banned from advertising altogether!

Since you don't have attorneys from the processed food industry standing over your shoulder, you don't have to be too rigorous with your definitions. They're really only crystallizations of your own understanding of these concepts.

Your definitions will be working definitions. That means you don't have to try to allow for all possible circumstances. Simply try to be clear and functional about expressing your *present* knowledge and feelings about the terms.

Undoubtedly, you have strong intuitive feelings for what is a natural food and what isn't. You have a feeling for what is a convenience food and what isn't. Your convenience food may be someone else's drudgery!

Notice I said "present" knowledge up above. Your knowledge, understanding, and feelings are going to grow and evolve. Keep this in mind when you assign value judgments.

There will be gray areas where definitions rely purely on feelings. For example, some people call all food that does not fit within their own value system for nutrition "junk food." I try to be more specific. I think of junk food as any food that is essentially worthless, made without concern for what food can and should be. To me, junk food includes mass-produced concoctions of artificial chemicals and other drastically altered substances. Junk food is designed to appeal to our less sophisticated tastes, while having minimal—or even negative— nutritional effects. Junk food is ill-conceived and executed. It began as junk and is better discarded as such.

A rich, natural pastry that a baker made by hand with the finest natural ingredients—in the wee hours before dawn so it would be fresh for the morning customers—may not be a nutritional gold mine, but I cannot call it junk. However, when a giant food conglomerate programs its computers to produce 5,000,000 Sugar Sponge Snack Cakes per month, load them into cellophane wrappers and ship them to supermarkets postdated two weeks down the line—*that* I call JUNK!

I find that when you get into the area of what is "good for you" and "bad for you," it's more effective to state differences in positive terms as much as possible. Be as descriptive as you can. Give your child plenty of examples. Don't just say, "This is bad for you, so you shouldn't eat it."

You may not even want to use the words "bad" or "wrong." You can say something like: "This food will help make you healthy and strong, but that other food won't. In fact that food might even cause you to feel sick."

Please Don't Be Dogmatic!

Please don't set yourself up for a situation in which you may later have to save face. Most people go through several stages in their natural foods revolution. They enter the natural foods "system" at one point with some ideas and plans about changing their diet. Then, as they get in deeper and read, talk, and experiment—and learn more about their own needs and responses—they find their ideas changing. Their awareness grows.

So please set up your system in such a way that you won't be uncomfortable with change. Don't ever feel you need to save face with your child over a change. One thing I find parents continually caught up in is saving face in front of their children.

It's a waste of energy. Make yourself human. You really can say to your child, "I was wrong. I made a mistake. I changed my mind. I know more now than I did then. I want to try something different."

You can set yourself and your child up for disappointment by straining to be superhuman and saying: "This is the only answer there is, so this is the way we're going to be doing it."

One of the best ways you can avoid this trap is by simply not making a big deal about your changes. Don't make rigid labels: "We're vegetarians." (Last year you were fructarians. What will you be next year?)

I know several people who have gone through these changes. They made the transitions more gracefully when they avoided putting labels on what they were doing. Instead, they placed themselves in the broad category of eating good, natural food. Then, any changes they made within that spectrum were easily accepted without fuss.

Children are not nearly as conservative as we adults sometimes make them out to be. They actually adapt themselves quite well—often better and more readily than adults. For seventeen years as a schoolteacher, I saw children successfully relate to many different teachers as they progressed from grade to grade.

It's fun to experiment and try new things. If you're careful not to be dogmatic and doctrinaire, you can express your growing involvement with natural foods in terms of a joyous new adventure. And if you're careful to maintain the important element of *we*, it's an adventure you and your child can share.

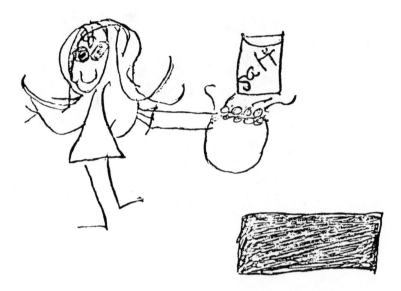

Be sure the rectangle is "black"

Japanese Rice Balls

Cook rice in a rice cooker. When it is done, put salt on it.

Put it in your hands and make a round ball.

Wrap it up in a black rectangle.

Kathy Tanji

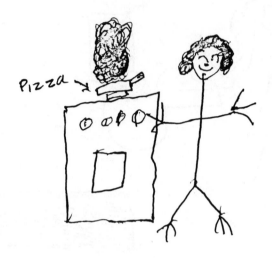

Pizza

For the dough you need ½ cup of flour. (This is a small pizza). Plop in 1 tablespoon of milk. Mix this up and dump it inside a plate. Put spaghetti and 2 teaspoons of spice on it.

Put it in the oven at 100° for 10 minutes. Take a toothpick and stick it in and then throw it away. (The tooth pick that is.)

This will serve a whole class.

Terry Yamamoto

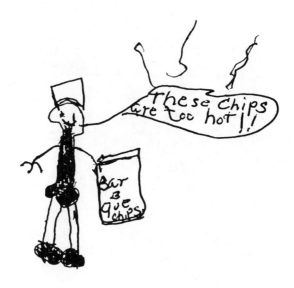

Bologna Sandwich

You need 2 pieces of white bread, mayonnaise, lettuce and 1 piece of bologna.

Put mayonnaise on 1 piece of bread. Put lettuce on, then the bologna and then the other junk. Put the other slice on.

Eat this with potato chips, but not the bar-b-que kind.

Dean Diaz

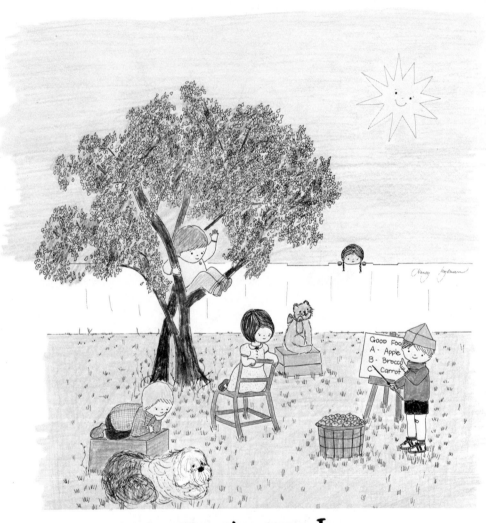

Teaching Is
An Act of Love

3

Think of yourself as a gardener. You are responsibile for this living growing person, this "seedling." Naturally, you want this young plant to thrive, and you want to provide it with all it needs to do that. One of those needs is good, nutritious food.

But there is another need your child depends on you for—a need you must keep in mind at all times, especially when trying to teach her something. This very basic need is one we all have. We need to love and accept ourselves.

This need has been expressed by many writers, but I like John Powell's description best: "One need so fundamental ... when met ... everything else will almost certainly harmonize in a general sense of well-being ... . When this need is properly nourished, the whole human organism will be healthy and the person will be happy. This need is true and deep love of self, a genuine and joyful self-acceptance, an authentic self-esteem, which results in an interior sense of celebration: 'It's good to be me!'"*

You, as parent, are, more than anyone else in the world, responsible for nourishing your child's self-esteem. A child can discover a lot about herself through her new experiences with food—just as she "learned" a lot when you fed her in response to her cries as an infant.

_____

*From *The Secret of Staying In Love*, p. 13, Argus Communications, Allen, Texas, 1974.

What we hope she will learn more of is that she is OK, she is lovable, and that it is good for her to be who she is.

Always try to strengthen your child's self-image. No one can be happy if this fundamental love of self is dampened or extinguished. Your efforts to teach your child about food *or anything else* will not succeed unless you show that you deeply believe she is—*without exception*—lovable and good.

If you challenge, attack, or fail to nurture your child's "inner celebration of self," she will be very unhappy, and the lesson of her unworthiness will be so strong that few positive lessons will ever be learned.

If your child's self-appreciation is damaged, her openness to *herself* will also be hampered. She will slowly lose the ability to be honest with herself—as well as with you and other people. If you put attention on policing where she goes wrong, your focused attention will indeed find faults. Your child's attention—and behavior—can always be counted on to go where your attention is.

So, look for positive things to praise and reward, rather than negative things to correct. Remember, you are the gardener. Where you shine the light, the plant will grow.

Make Yourself Vulnerable

Since your child is so vulnerable to you, try to make yourself vulnerable to her. To do this you may have to turn yourself around to a new way of thinking. Do you think that a parent is an all-powerful, all-knowing being who must make all decisions for a child until she is eighteen, twenty-one, thirty-three, or perhaps a grandparent? If you do, please reconsider! This attitude puts you in a position in which it's almost impossible to admit a mistake. You waste a lot of energy constantly defending your infallibility, and you put yourself at odds with your child. You wind up defending your own "rightness" at the expense of hers.

So, climb down out of the fort and make yourself vulnerable to your child. Start by incorporating and respecting her viewpoint. Because she is so vulnerable to you, think about what feelings towards her are expressed through your actions. Do your actions demonstrate to her that she is worthy of love? Do they demonstrate that you really enjoy being with her? Do they demonstrate that you feel relaxed or ill at ease when she wants to interrupt a conversation or just enter a room and be with you?

Do your actions demonstrate that you look forward with enthusiasm to being with her? Or do they demonstrate that she is an irritant and you can hardly wait for her to grow up and leave home?

Do your actions demonstrate that you enthusiastically celebrate your child's existence?

What do your actions demonstrate?

I know ... sometimes we're not totally in control of what our actions demonstrate. Sometimes we feel we need to put love aside for a moment and do "what has to be done." And sometimes we just don't know *how* to let love pass between us and our children.

It's times like this we would like to have a road map, a set of principles to guide us. We want to keep our end of the bargain—and we want our child to do the same.

As I assembled my thoughts and notes for this book, I found that my suggestions were guided by certain basic principles. Looking back over my experience as a teacher and a mother, I saw that these principles had not only guided me, but also *supported* me. When I honestly felt that I didn't know what to do, I could fall back on them for direction and guidance.

When I was confused, I could sort out my emotions by testing what I *felt like doing* against what I *knew* would actually bring me closer to my goals.

I am putting these six principles all together in one place so you can easily review them. They are:

Acceptance

Responsibility

Freedom

Honesty

Affirmation

Fun

These six words represent acts on your part. Test your attitudes and actions against them. It's often too easy to justify what we, as parents and teachers, do by saying "because I love you."

"I'm yelling at you because I love you!"

"I'm grounding you for a month because I love you."

"I forbid you to climb that tree because I love you."

"I'm forcing you to go to law school because I love you."

"I'm forbidding you to eat Greaseburgers and Fatty-fries because I love you!"

"Eat these bean sprouts because I love you!"

We act out of several emotions—not just love. We can be angry, and act out of anger, but we often justify the act out of love, because we feel love, too. So to say, "I'm doing this because I love you" isn't always a tough enough test. We've all found that "because I love you" doesn't always work the kind of magic we expect of love. The words alone don't always clear the way.

But these six principles are tough and strong. It's tougher to be able to say, "I'm doing this because I *accept* you." You can see right away if what you're doing really says you accept your child.

"I want you to choose the color for your new shirt, because I respect your freedom."

"I'm not punishing you after you have told me you ate a half dozen Greaseburgers, because it's more important that we be honest with each other."

"I want you to cook that meal yourself because I want you to learn responsibility."

These six principles can help you teach your child. They are avenues for love, which is a two-way street.

Acceptance

When you accept a child, you help him validate himself. You nourish his self-image rather than attack or diminish it. You let him know you believe he is absolutely wonderful!

I learned the value of acceptance and validation when I was a teacher. The lesson was really brought home to me when I taught Head Start children in nursery school and kindergarten. These children were very young and their vocabulary was limited, so they could not express themselves very well. I learned to pay close attention to their facial expressions and moods to gauge how well they were responding.

I realized that when I treated children with acceptance and a positive attitude, I got a better response. They smiled and opened their eyes wide in excitement or narrowed them in curious concentration.

In later years, when teaching older children, I had more to go on than facial expressions and moods. I had standardized test scores— which were always phenomenal. My students' scores were the best in the district year after year (for the grade I was teaching).

There was a good reason for that success. The children really wanted to learn. It was fun for them. They knew I believed they were wonderful.

If you praise a child, if you always increase his self-esteem rather than decrease it, he'll jump at the chance to join you. If he gains in self-confidence by learning, he'll eagerly open himself up to what you have to teach.

Go into any good classroom, and you'll see this taking place. You will see children learning because they are validated for their accomplishments. They are never made to feel fundamentally "wrong."

When they make a mistake, they are encouraged to feel that they can and will do better. They always know they have a chance to go back and correct it. Their mistakes do not diminish either their teacher's acceptance of them or their own self-acceptance.

Accept your child and don't let anything get in the way of that acceptance. Don't let anything block the communication that lets him know you accept him. Remember, his deepest need is to believe that he is lovable and valuable and acceptable just by virtue of *being*.

Responsibility

There is a Chinese proverb that says we forget what we hear, remember what we see, and understand what we *do*. I heartily subscribe to that proverb. Our children learn best when they get in there and do whatever it is we want them to learn.

Giving your child responsibility means many things. It means involving her in cooking, shopping, and decision making. It means allowing her to learn by experience as well as by discussion, by action as well as by thought.

What does the word itself say about what we want? We want her to be *responsible* and take on *responsibilities*. Then, it seems right to me that we must encourage her to *respond* to her successes as well as her mistakes.

A child needs to feel that she is contributing to her family and to the people around her. She cannot develop into a healthy, productive individual unless there is a back and forth flow of expectations, achievement, and satisfaction. Your praise of her accomplishments is nutrition-packed food for her growing self-esteem and confidence.

Encourage her to develop responsibility gradually and consistently by giving her tasks that you know she can do. Then gradually raise your expectations.

For example, you may expect your four year old son to help you knead the bread dough. After he has mastered that, you can add another task in the baking process—such as pouring in the honey and water.

By performing tasks that are valuable to the whole family, he will develop self-image building relationships with other family members. For example, you may expect him to perform simple household chores such as picking up the toys in his room. Then, once he has mastered that, add another task such as setting the table or feeding the pets.

Ultimately, we want our children to set their own goals in life and achieve them. You can help your child develop self-motivation by sitting down with him and agreeing on what his goals and responsibilities will be for the chores and other activities. Give him a choice of several alternatives, if possible. Then, as your expectations rise, so will his— immeasurably strengthening his inner sense of strength and power.

I know that one of the hardest things for some parents to do is "let go" and allow their children to try something on their own. When you're teaching your child to ride a bicycle, for example, it really hurts to remove your hands from the bike and let the child go.

Yet we all have to do it sooner or later. Perhaps in our hearts we never let go, but we all must allow our children to ride off, even if we are always ready and willing to jump back and be there for them if they need us. I thank God my father was ready, willing, and able to jump back and put his steadying hands on the bicycle for me, long after I had ridden off as an adult.

Freedom

We've all heard the statement, "There is no freedom without responsibility" pronounced as if it were a curse of some kind. To me, the fact that freedom and responsibility go hand in hand is a joyful reality, not a grim necessity. I feel happy when I think that there is no responsibility without freedom. Our expectations for our children can be guided by an equal commitment to their freedom.

After all, our children are not our possessions. We should not assume that they want to be or *should* want to be exactly as we would like.

I know a young man who wanted to be an artist, but his parents didn't want him to have to struggle to make a good living the way they had, so they forced him to go to law school. It took him five years to get through law school, when most students finish in three. When he finally graduated, his parents bought him a lucrative practice from a retiring attorney. Now, however, the practice is no longer thriving. The young man is struggling to make ends meet.

His parents, though they loved him, ignored one fact. It's one thing to be doing what you want to do and struggle for success, but it's another to struggle in bondage to something you don't really want to do.

Honesty

It's wonderful when your child feels free to tell you *anything*. It's vital that the lines of communication between you and your child be maintained freely flowing.

Don't let the apparent simplicity of this principle fool you. There will be times when your daughter has "bad news." At these times, remember that if you punish her after she has told you about a mistake, she will not learn to stop making the mistake. She will learn to stop telling you.

Honesty is a kind of freedom. When you are honest, you are free to express what you see, feel, and believe. When there is honesty between people, there is a free flow of vital communication, which every relationship needs to remain healthy and constructive. One of the most important benefits we receive from a close relationship is the freedom to share ourselves with someone—to share *all* information about ourselves, too.

Affirmation

The area upon which we focus the light of our attention is the area that will experience the most growth or activity. Think of your attention as being a very powerful source of energy. If you direct it at negative things, you will strengthen them in your mind and in your child's mind. You will make it harder, not easier, to prevent further errors and encourage growth.

On the other hand, if you direct your attention to positive things, you will strengthen them in your mind and in your child's mind and make it easier for them to win out.

Affirm the positive things your son can do. Focus attention on his accomplishments and suggest new ones for the future. By praising his ability you will reinforce his desire to achieve. His sense of confidence and acceptance will grow, because you are making him right and good. You are, in effect, saying to him: "These things you can do are wonderful! You can grow and get better all the time! Wow! Isn't that wonderful?"

It *is* wonderful, because that's exactly what he will do.

Positive affirmation means looking for the best in life and going after it.

Fun

Give your child good memories with good food. If we strive to be relaxed, cheerful, and comfortable when preparing and serving food, a bright spirit of celebration can grace our activities. We can make mealtimes happy, peaceful, nourishing times.

Our involvement with food, from the shopping to the eating, doesn't have to be drudgery. We can do whatever we need to do in order to make these activities fun. Every meal can be a celebration. No meal has to be automatic or mechanical.

I am not suggesting that you get out balloons and streamers for every meal, but there's no reason you have to reserve them for birthdays and New Year's Eve! You can take every opportunity for enjoyment that exists around food and meals.

You can perform all of the lessons and activities in this book in the spirit of adventure and fun. We all learn best—and do our best—when it's fun.

I was discussing these six principles with a friend recently. My friend had a guest along, and, after listening for a while, the guest—who had no children—wondered out loud whether "all of this wonderful acceptance and freedom and fun might not spoil a child."

My friend, who has three teenage children, answered for me: "Oh, not at all. You don't spoil a child when you give too much love. Only when you don't give enough."

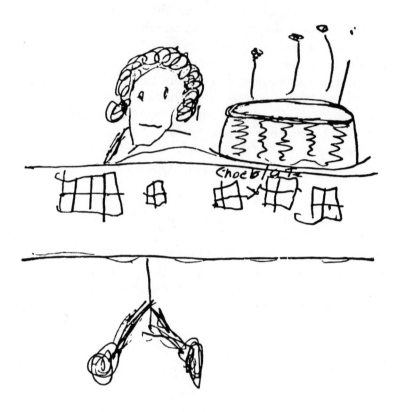

Chocolate Cake

Put pie dough in the pan. Put the pan in a real
hot oven. Take out the pan. Make the icing with 4
cups of milk, 10 packs of chocolate and 5 cups of
sugar. Cook this on the stove for 30 hours. Pour
the icing on the cake *softly*. Then, cook the cake
for 30 hours in the oven. Take it out and leave it
alone for a few minutes.

Gregg Thompson

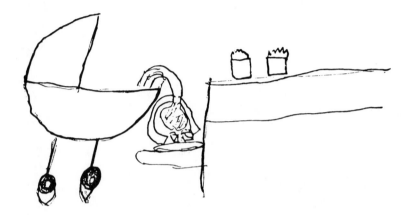

Cupcakes

You need a bunch of stuff in the bowl. Stir it around with a thing and put all this in the refrigerator. Leave it awhile and then pour it into some small paper things. Pop this in a 40° oven. Take them out and frost them.

Now, put them back in the oven so the baby won't get any!

Roger Goss

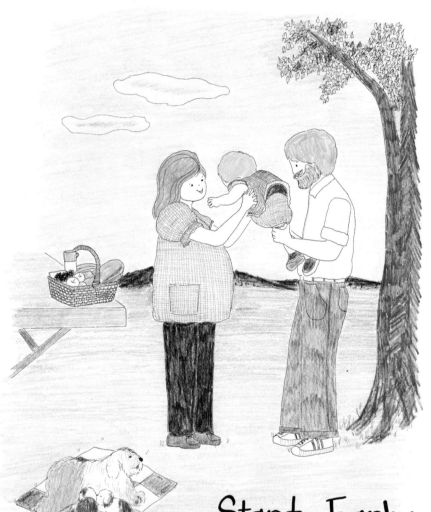

Start Early

4

It's true that you can change your child's diet for the better no matter how old he is. But the earlier you start, the easier it will be.

I know that you may be reading this book for help in changing the diets of children already beyond infancy. I include this brief section not only for those who may be just starting—or adding to—a family, but also to stay true to my conviction that it's never too late—or too early—to improve your child's health with natural foods.

We've known for years that poor diet, cigarette smoking, and consumption of alcohol and coffee can harm an unborn child. Medical research has also found that a mother and father's diet *before conception* can also affect the health of a soon-to-be conceived child. And it's only very recently that we've learned that these habits can influence an unborn child's psychological and physical relations with food and other substances *later in life*.

A hypnotherapist friend and I were talking about this one evening, when he told me something fascinating. While working with people who have compulsions for alcohol, cigarettes, and other drugs, he often uses a process called hypnotic regression. His patients are hypnotically taken back in their memories to try to locate the moments when there were physical or emotional events that helped create their compulsions. In most cases, the moment in time is during early childhood. But in an amazing number of cases, the hypnotist is able to take them *all the way back to moments in the womb when alcohol or nicotine entered their bloodstream!*

39

Feed Your Baby the Natural Way

Starting early to keep your end of the bargain also means feeding your baby natural food right from the moment of birth. The best natural food you can feed your baby is, of course, mother's milk. The benefits of breast feeding and the disadvantages of processed formula feeding are many.

Breast-fed babies are protected against a long list of diseases. They are less likely to suffer from: dehydration, meningitis, asthma, hives, eczema, high blood pressure, dermatitis, growth retardation, hypocalcemic tetany, neonatal hypothyroidism, Sudden Infant Death Syndrome, learning disorders, colitis, malocclusion, colon cancer, iron deficiency anemia, allergies, food sensitivities, nursing bottle caries, gastroenteritis, pneumonia, otitis media, recurrent colds, bronchitis, colic, diarrhea, vomiting, abdominal pain syndrome, hyperactive-type disturbances of behavior (as a consequence of allergy to cow's milk), septicemia, hyponatremia, and acrodermatitis enteropathica (zinc deficiency).

Mother's milk is loaded with several vital factors that arm a baby's immune system against invading disease organisms and other harmful substances. Breast milk boosts every element of a baby's defenses, including protection from diseases to which mother and baby have recently been exposed. The mother's immune system actually does the work the baby's immature system cannot—by manufacturing immunity factors and passing them to baby through the milk.

The earliest atherosclerotic changes in blood vessels occur not in middle-aged men, but in babies fed processed artificial formula. Breast-fed infants have been found to handle cholesterol and other fats better than formula-fed infants *later in life*, too.

The old adage, "You never see a fat breast-fed baby" may be true. Breast-fed babies do seem to have less of a problem with obesity when they are children and when they are grown up. Formula feeding and early introduction of high-calorie solid food play havoc with an infant's developing ability to self-regulate his food intake. This can drastically affect eating habits later in life.

Feeding highly sweetened foods to babies during infancy has been linked not only to obesity, but also to diabetes, diverticular disease, and colon cancer.

Many of the health problems breast feeding appears to protect against are no doubt caused by the nutritional inadequacies of processed infant formulas. Formula has been called everything from the "first junk food" to "baby's first drug." (In fact, the top three processed formulas *are manufactured by* drug companies!)

Processed infant formulas are hardly natural foods. On the contrary, processed formula epitomizes the arrogance of the food industry. It's man-made by so-called "experts" who sometimes goof— and then is heavily promoted to replace an inexpensive, convenient, vastly superior natural food.

Any baby who is formula fed is vulnerable not only to gaps in the "experts'" knowledge, but also to the usual errors and oversights that are to be expected with any highly-processed, manufactured food.

In the early 1950s, thousands of parents across the country were terrified when their babies inexplicably went into convulsions. Doctors were mystified, too, until one of them observed that the convulsions stopped when the infants' formula was changed. Further investigation revealed that a major formula manufacturer had—through a "new, improved" process—inadvertantly produced formula without one vital ingredient: vitamin B6. This error and some more recent industrial mistakes have left several innocent babies deformed, retarded, or impaired for life.

The nutritional contents of mother's milk are balanced for the needs of a human baby. These balances are widely different in the milk of various animals. Cow's milk, for example, has too much protein and salt for a human baby's system to handle. This imbalance puts a strain on a baby's kidneys. The protein in human milk, however, contains all the right amino acids in the right balance, so it's easier to digest. The iron in mother's milk is easier to absorb, too.

Breast feeding has psychological and emotional advantages, too. Breast feeding encourages "bonding." The breast-fed infant can hear his mother's heartbeat much of the time he is nursing. The close, warm bodily contact establishes a fundamental sense of trust and security in the baby. Studies have found that this mother-child interaction results in a more complex and satisfying relationship between mother and child later in life.

All during my pregnancy, I looked forward to nursing my newborn child, but when Kristin was born, I came down with a serious infection. Massive doses of drugs were required. While I was on the drugs, I was not able to nurse Kristin.

When the infection was gone, I anxiously waited until all traces of the drugs had disappeared from my milk, and then I tried nursing Kristin. I tried and tried, but my milk just wouldn't come in the quantities necessary to adequately nourish my daughter. I had to give up.

For me, it was a tragic disappointment. I can empathize with mothers who are not able to nurse their infants. I also appreciate the growing awareness and skills fostered by the La Leche League, an international organization with local chapters. Founded more than a quarter century ago by seven mothers and now more than 1.25 million members strong, the League encourages, supports, and teaches about breast feeding. I heartily recommend this organization as a source of information and support.

My disappointing experience proves the value of taking the best care of yourself that you can. If I had done that, I may have avoided the infection and resulting drug treatment that prevented me from nursing my daughter.

Thankfully, for mothers who are not able to breast feed their babies, there are now natural alternatives to chemically-processed infant formula. One natural alternative is to purchase mother's milk from women who are producing more than their infants need. The La Leche League can advise you on how to go about purchasing breast milk.

There are other natural alternatives to processed formula. There are formulas that utilize blends of natural ingredients such as grains and goat's milk, which is much closer to human milk in nutritional composition than cow's milk.

There is one such formula that has been used for infant feeding for more than 2000 years. It utilizes barley water, milk (cow's or goat's), and a natural sweetener (maple syrup is the preferred, since honey may be difficult for young infants to digest). This recipe is given on the following page.

One of the benefits of this formula is that the enzymes in the barley water soften the milk curds and make the cow's milk easier for the baby to digest. There is a powdered, natural form of this formula, called NaturLac, available from Steve Lederman, Sunrise and Rainbow, 9526 Pico Blvd., Suite 5, Los Angeles, Calif. 90035, 213-276-7237.

Formula-fed infants tend to suffer from colic more often than breast-fed babies, but for all babies suffering from colic, there are natural alternatives to the drugs doctors often prescribe. These natural remedies include:

1. lactobacillus acidophilus culture, which can be purchased in powdered or liquid form and added to the formula. ("Megadophilus" is a very potent and reliable acidophilus culture. It was developed by and is available from Natasha Trenev, 12142 Huston Street, North Hollywood, Calif. 91607, 213-761-0044.)

2. two herbs which have been used for centuries to treat colic—catnip and hops tea.

When your child is weaned, you can chop, grind, mash, blend, puree—and feed him—the same wonderfully wholesome and nutritious natural foods the rest of your family enjoys.

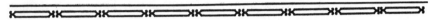

Infant Formula

15 ounces barley water
10 ounces milk (goat's or cow's)
1-2 tablespoons maple syrup (natural maple syrup, not imitation!)

To make barley water, place approximately one cup of pearled barley in a cheese cloth, and tie it so that the barley can't get out in the water. Be sure to tie it loosely to allow room for the barley to expand. Place the cheese cloth with the barley in a large stainless steel pot. (*Don't use aluminum!*) Pour in two quarts of water. Bring to a boil, and then turn the heat down to simmer. Simmer for six hours so that all of the nutritional elements from the barley can be absorbed into the water. Keep an eye on the water now and then so that as the water evaporates, you can add more. The water will turn pink. In the end, you want at least fifteen ounces of barley water, which will make a day's serving when added to the milk and maple syrup. At the end of six hours, discard the cheese cloth with the cooked barley. You will have to start over with fresh barley the next time you make the formula. (You can use the cooked barley in soups, casseroles, or for breakfast, if you wish.)

Mix the barley water in a container with the milk and maple syrup. Pour the formula in four eight-ounce sterilized bottles and store in the refrigerator until used (within 48 hours). At feeding time, warm the water to body temperature.

Starting early to keep your end of the natural foods bargain with your child may lead you into some new and exciting adventures. When Rondi and Rich Prescott's baby started cutting teeth, little did they know that their commitment to a totally natural foods diet for their baby would lead them into a whole new career!

Rondi—who majored in nutrition at Colorado State University—went on a quest for a natural teething biscuit. She couldn't find one anywhere, so she decided to make her own. She mixed up a favorite recipe for molasses cookies (whole wheat flour, nonfat dry milk powder, unsulphured molasses, and wheat germ), and left it out overnight to dry. The next morning she shaped them with the only cookie cutter she had—a heart shape—and baked them. The result: natural teething biscuits! And heart-shaped to boot!

Some days later, Rondi took her baby to a wholistic pediatrician for a checkup. The baby had one of the teething biscuits, which the pediatrician noticed. He remarked that he knew dozens of mothers who would love to have such a wonderful biscuit for their babies.

The rest is history. "Healthy Times" (4835 Voltaire Street, Suite 107, San Diego, Calif. 92107) now produces natural teething biscuits by the thousands, and sells them to natural foods stores throughout the country.

Rondi's and Rich's story demonstrates how resourceful a family that's making a commitment to a natural foods diet can be. That resourcefulness may not pay off with a growing business for everyone, but the real bottom line—your family's health—will thrive.

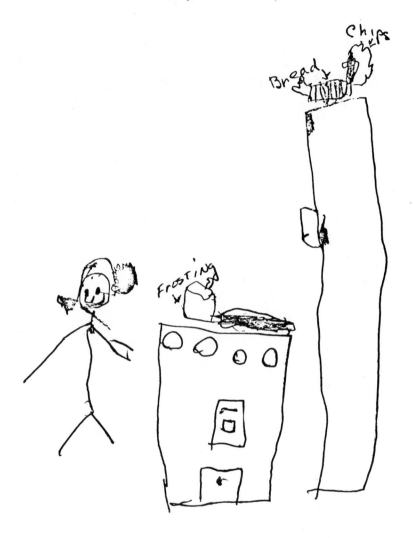

Chocolate Cake

You need chocolate, 2 eggs, 1 bag of flour and 1 bag of sugar. Mix it together with a blender. The oven is hot as a fire.

Take it out and put frosting on the cake and put it back in the oven so the frosting will stick to the cake.

Michelle Novis

Nutrition From

to

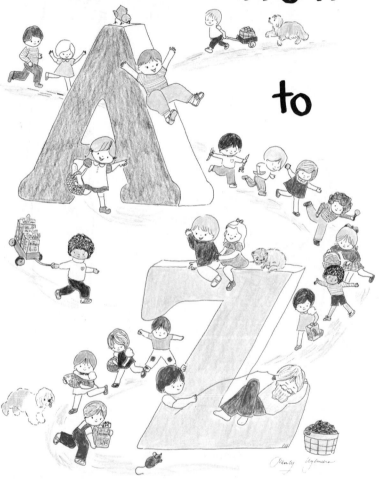

For Kids 1 to 100

5

Jane knows nutrition backwards and forwards. She is a registered nurse, has had college nutrition courses, and has studied therapeutic nutrition with some of the best teachers. When I talked to her not very long ago, she was having a problem with her seven year old daughter, Annie.

"I'm trying to teach Annie some of the basics of nutrition," Jane said. "Simple concepts. What vitamins do. What protein does. But Annie won't cooperate! I sit down and talk to her about biochemical reactions, but she seems bored. When I ask her about the lessons later on, she doesn't remember very much at all. I even try to meet her halfway by using words she should understand!"

"Janie," I said, "you have to go a whole lot further than meeting Annie halfway. You have to go *all the way*! Teach on *her* terms.

"Annie's only been here seven years. She's a newcomer! The world is a big adventure to her. She came into it eager to explore, but she can't do it all at once. It's too much! She has tons of curiosity, but her young mind can't grapple with everything that goes on.

"Her capacity for learning will expand, but it takes time. As it grows, you need to put your information into shapes and sizes that can fit into her mind."

We all want our children to "see things our way." We want them to prefer wheat germ to bubble gum, yogurt to popsicles, orange juice to cola. We also want them to make these choices using the same information we use.

But something goes wrong when we try to give them that information. We suddenly feel as if we're speaking a foreign language. They just can't—or won't—"see things our way." So maybe we push a little harder. Or we talk slower. Or louder. Or we talk *more*.

That can be a big mistake. To get a child to "see things our way" is usually impossible, and pushing too hard assaults the child's self-esteem. You see, a child's sense of reality is rooted in her point of view—in *her* way of seeing things.

To make her see things our way, we would have to first take apart her way.

Or ... we might just try to heap our fertile wisdom on her to try to make her awareness grow faster.

If that didn't work, we might criticize her as "dumb" or "childish." We might just get a little angry and grab hold of her sense of reality and self-esteem and try to shake some sense into it.

If we chose any one of these approaches, we would be attacking the very center of her reality. To try to push her beyond her reasoning and conceptual powers would not only frustrate her, but would also make her feel unworthy, powerless, and stupid.

She can't be pushed. She must take the steps herself.

When a young child sees a flying squirrel, she'll most likely call it a bird. She doesn't yet have a place in her view of reality for mammals that fly. If you try to squeeze the flying squirrel in, you may wind up distorting her view of reality. Or ... at the very least, you may bore and confuse her. To comfortably—and effectively—fit that flying squirrel into her view of reality, you need to meet your child on her mind's level of development—and take the flying squirrel with you.

The French scientist Piaget designed several vivid experiments to demonstrate the different developmental levels a child's reasoning powers pass through on the way to adulthood. The most famous of these experiments is one in which two identical vessels of water are placed before a child. Because both vessels are transparent, it's easy to see that both hold equal amounts of water. Any child, at any age or developmental level, would be able to point that out.

Next, two empty vessels are brought in. These, however, are not identical in shape, but they do hold the same amount of water. One vessel is tall and slender, the other short and fat.

The first, identical vessels are then emptied into the second vessels—in full view of the child. Now, the tall, slender vessel will have a tall column of water reaching almost to the top. The short, fat vessel will also be nearly full.

At this point, if you ask the child which vessel has more water in it, you will get a different answer, depending on the child's developmental level. A child in either of what Piaget called the "sensorimotor" (birth to 18 months) or the "preoperational" (18 months to 7 years) stages will probably say that the taller vessel has more water. A child in either the "concrete operational" (7 to 12 years) or "formal operational" (12 years to adult) stage will say that both vessels still have equal amounts of water. (It's not necessary to remember Piaget's names for these levels. Nor is it necessary to consider the age brackets as one hundred percent accurate in every child. They are only approximate.)

Are you beginning to see why you need to meet your child on her own terms? You need to tune in to her developmental level before she'll understand you. You can perform Piaget's experiment before a four year old, then demonstrate how the same amount of water is going into both vessels. You can jump up and down, cajole, yell, and bribe—and maybe get her to nod her head and say, "Yes, there is the same amount of water in both." But deep down, where it counts, she will not believe it. You may get your child to repeat or memorize something, but her real "learning center" will only hang on to the concepts she can grasp—and only in a form that will fit into her scheme of things.

Your child must make a mental picture of what you are saying or demonstrating before she can learn, and children simply do not have the same pictures in their minds as you or I normally do. You must present an acceptable "mind picture" that will convey the correct message. Build that picture first in your own mind, and then present it to your child a piece at a time.

A child's mind is very selective. It filters out of consciousness many stimuli she can't understand or relate to. Children, after all, really aren't concerned with many of the things we adults are. So it's necessary to go to their world of interests to find impressions, concerns, and pictures that they will be able to approach with ease, pleasure, curiosity,and excitement.

For example, to try to bring home to a three year old the idea that natural food will help you live a long life, is a waste of time. Most three year olds do not have a concept of long or short life. Three year olds "know" they are going to live forever.

On the other hand, if you demonstrate to a three year old that natural foods are more fun to prepare and eat, you'll be in business.

The following two chapters are designed to help you approach your child with a combination of discussion, demonstration, and active participation that will help you reach her level. Each chapter consists of a discussion of the fundamentals of nutrition followed by several activities you can do together.

In these teaching chapters, I will try to give you a strong foundation. As you build on this foundation and teach your child more and more about nutrition, the chapters that come later will help you deal with the challenges, frustrations, and brickbats that come your way.

Although each of those later chapter has its own plan for discussion and activities, you may still want to refer back to these teaching chapters—

When your children are hooked on Bonzo the Clown's Artificial Brownies and you want to explain why natural snacks are better ...

When your mate or your parents or the schoolteacher shrug their shoulders and exclaim: "But how do you explain these things to kids?"

When you've succeeded in helping your children tune out TV advertising but now need some good news to put in its place ...

And any of the thousand and one times you may want to explain some aspect of nutrition to someone between the ages of 1 and 100!

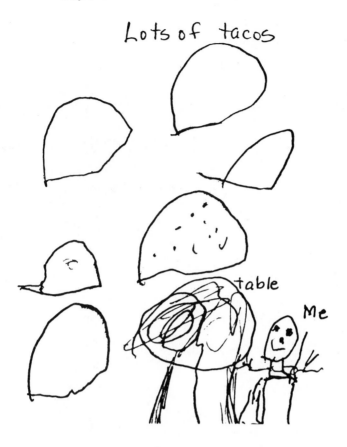

Lots of tacos

table

Me

Tacos

First, you get a pan. Then put butter in it. Then, put oil in the pan. Pour both of these out. Put on the lid. Put in a taco and cook it. Cook a pack of meat in oil and cook and cook it. Turn it over with a thing and mash it all up. Put the meat in the taco. Put on ketchup and sliced cheese. Get a paper towel and wrap it up on the outside of the taco.

Eat it with your hands because it is really simple that way.

Michael Miller

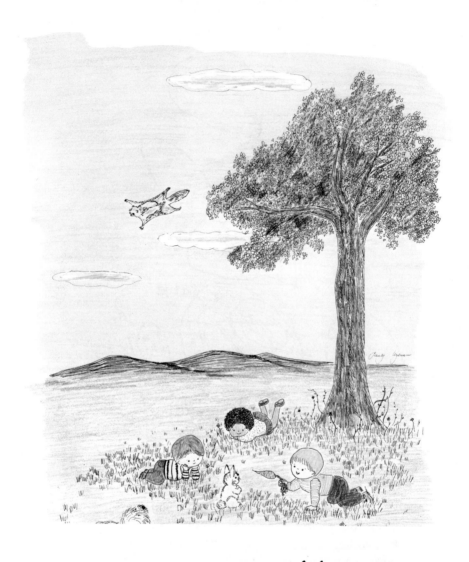

A Vitamin
Is Like A Flying Squirrel

6

Up to the age of seven, a child is limited in his ability to build "mind pictures" of some of the fundamentals of nutrition. You will have to work carefully to go the extra distance to meet him on his level, which means your mind pictures will have to be simple ones.

Don't let this discourage you. The simplicity of the young child's view of reality works in your favor. A child this young will be extremely cooperative. He'll do whatever you do. You can spend hours making up entertaining stories about how wonderful natural foods can be, but the chances are good that he'll learn to prefer natural foods more from what you feed him than from what you tell him.

That doesn't mean the young child can't learn some important facts about nutrition, too. If you follow the six principles in Chapter 3, and if you're careful to work in tune with his view of the world, your young child can grasp an amazing amount of fundamental information. He does, however, have certain limitations you should be aware of.

A young child doesn't have what Piaget called "conservation." When he sees the water poured into a different-shaped container, he does not see in his mind that the amount of water is the same in both containers. He cannot visualize that the water is the same—that it was conserved, and merely transferred from one container to another. He cannot visualize the reverse operation, either—pouring the water back into the first container—unless it actually takes place.

Children this young tend to see and think in absolute terms. They don't understand such concepts as "more," "equal," "darker," "longer," "larger," "better," and "healthier," the way adults do. Even relational terms such as "right," "left," "brother," and "sister," are seen in very subjective ways. A young child may know *his* brother as "brother," but may balk at accepting that someone else can have a "brother," too.

In another of Piaget's experiments, a young child was shown two rows of seven identical buttons. One row was spaced so that it was longer than the other. The child was asked to count the number of buttons in each row, which he did correctly. He was then asked which row had *more* buttons.

The child insisted that the longer row had more buttons!

Can you imagine what might happen if you tried to explain to a four year old that whole wheat bread was "better" because it had "more" of what was "good" for him? He might learn to choose the *longest* loaf of bread he could find!

A child this young may have difficulty drawing a picture in his mind of a series of actions, even if he knows every action and can follow the sequence. He can learn what turns to make in order to find his way to his friend's house five blocks away, but if you asked him to draw a map to his friend's house, he couldn't do it. Keep this in mind when you are trying to explain a concept such as the food chain in nature, or a sequence such as digestion.

A child at this developmental level also has difficulty reasoning about things as parts of a whole. He sees things absolutely, as they relate to him. Likewise, he cannot visualize in his mind things he can't see with his eyes.

To try to make a child this young grasp the chemistry of vitamins, proteins, carbohydrates, and fats would be futile. Any correct picture you might try to draw of these concepts would not represent anything the child could *see*, so it wouldn't be real to him. This is also true of bodily processes with which he has no conscious connection, such as the manufacture of red blood cells in the bone marrow, the exchange of oxygen and waste products between the blood and the cells, and other metabolic reactions. If we want to get our ideas across, we must relate them to what he can see.

What are some of the things your child likes to do? What are the sensations and situations he takes note of and tells you about? Does he like to run, skip, jump, climb, swim, or ride a bicycle?

Observe the important activities in his life and help him make the association between them and nutrition. For example, if he enjoys riding his bicycle (or tricycle), you can explain that the whole wheat bread he loves to eat *helps* him enjoy that activity by giving him the energy to do it.

I must caution you. Don't go too far with the association. Otherwise, the child may get the idea that eating enormous amounts of the food will give him super strength and endurance.

You can explain the difference between being out of energy because of hunger and because of exhaustion: "Sometimes we run out of energy and feel tired and hungry, but sometimes we're just plain tired and need to rest."

You don't have to *lecture* your child about any of these things. Just talk about them in a relaxed manner when you're handling or preparing food.

Try these questions:

What is food?"

("Food is whatever I eat. Food is what tastes good!")

"Where does food come from?"

("From the stove. From the refrigerator. From Mommy. From the car in brown bags Daddy carries in. From the market.")

"Why do we eat?"

("Because we're hungry. Because it tastes good. Because Grandma came over and brought dessert.")

"What is a healthy body?"

("When you don't get sick!" "What does 'healthy' mean, Mommy?")

The answers to all these questions can easily be connected to a young child's world. Food, to him, is whatever he eats. Use this very simple fact as a jumping off point. You can ask him to make a list of what he eats, if not in writing then in pictures he can draw himself. Have him name the foods. If any of them are at hand, show them to him.

As you are talking about or handling the food, let the positive, cheerful tone of your voice communicate to him that the food is "good." From this point, you can eventually make a very important connection.

First, explore how the food relates to the earth by asking him, "Where does the food come from?" Lead him back from the concrete, specific items of food that are vivid parts of his immediate world to the earth, which is the source of all food.

"Yes, the food comes out of the brown bags Daddy brings home from the market, but before they get to the market, they come from ... a farm." At this point, you can show him photographs of farms, animals, crops, fishing boats, etc. to give him a picture of the source of the food. Try to show him that all real food comes from living things.

Next, ask him, "Why do we eat food? What does food do for us?"

Remember to talk about food in terms of activities he experiences regularly. You might say something like, "Food helps us to be strong. Food helps us grow. Food helps us get better when we're sick."

You can even associate specific activities with specific foods, but be careful not to confuse him with concepts that are too abstract or sophisticated. For example, when he's eating an orange, you can say, "Oranges help keep us from getting sick."

You can mention vitamin C and his immune system, but remember: Vitamins are like flying squirrels. Chances are they'll fly right over his view of the world at this stage.

Remember our principle of affirmation. Most of the associations you make about food and health should be positive. Your child is very vulnerable to your value judgments at this age. When you make your associations, do it gently.

You can get into the concept that some foods are better than others by using the associations you have already set up. Food comes from living things and helps us do what we enjoy. Foods that are damaged in factories or foods that have chemicals added to them that don't come from living things *don't help as much*. Establish in his mind the simple connections between living food and the adventures of his life.

When some food is clearly junk, you can identify it as such and he will get the message. At this point, don't try to give him the notion that Purple Chemi-Doo-Dads will "hurt" him. He may then expect to see his friends who eat them writhing in pain. When he doesn't see that happen, he may begin to doubt you.

You can simply tell him that junk food does not do the wonderful things that living food does. Show your own sincere distaste for junk food through your facial expressions and the tone of your voice.

"Yecccch! (grimace) Sugar Rockets are junk!"

Take a Trip to a Farm

Here's your chance to really expand your child's "mind picture" of food. I've never known a young child who didn't enjoy a visit to a farm. There's no better way to impress upon him where food comes from than to actually take him there and show him. Let him see, smell, hear, and touch the animals, plants, and earth. Let him see that food comes from living animals and plants—not out of a box.

Most of us are still fortunate enough to live within a short drive of a real farm. If a trip to a farm is out of the question right now, find some way to come as close to the real thing as possible. Show your child photographs of farms. Take him beyond the pictures by talking about or reading stories about life on the farm. You can find books and articles about farming at the library. Perhaps you can even find a movie or TV show that will feature a real farm.

Naturally, the more involved the child can get in the farm the better. But even stopping on the side of the road and getting out to experience cows, chickens, turkeys, ducks, geese, or pigs that are on the other side of the fence can be a good lesson.

Enrich the experience any way you can. Take a camera and/or a tape recorder with you. Bring home as many sensations and mementoes as you can.

Sue Epstein, who was Director of Nutrition at Mrs. Gooch's for six years, told me this story about the wonderful experience she and her grandchildren had when they lived together in rural Germany for a year:

"The youngest was eighteen months old. The oldest was four years old. My daughter was at work most of the day, so Grandma—yours truly—got the babies. They both had virtually no experience with natural foods, so I made it a fun experience for them.

"I involved them in making everything from granola to yogurt, and we didn't just drive to a supermarket for milk. We went to the farms for our groceries. I had a baby under one arm, a gallon jug under the other—with the four year old tugging at my skirt as we piled into the Volkswagen for our excursion to the farms.

"Three miles away from where we lived, there was a little

farm. They had a small barn with only enough room for half a dozen cows. Their milking machine was a tiny gas engine affair that could milk only one cow at a time as it went 'chugachug chugachug chugachug.'

"And the farmer's wife loved us because we didn't speak very much German and she didn't speak very much English. She would pick up the children and carry them into the barn and have them pet the cows. We'd get our gallon jug filled with fresh milk and climb back into the little car.

"Then we'd drive to the next farm, where the children would help gather eggs right out of the nests.

"The children learned a lot during that wonderful year. They had milk right from the cow, eggs right out of the nest, and vegetables right out of the ground. Twice a week we'd go to an open-air market—rain, shine, or snow. The farmers put umbrellas over their tables and little gas heaters in their booths. There was a warm feeling of camaraderie and caring that we all shared. I know the children really benefited from it, too. Both grandchildren and my daughter learned a lot about food. Since then, natural foods have been a very big part of their way of life."

Shopping

Take advantage of many different kinds of shopping experiences: supermarkets, natural food markets, co-ops, "Mom and Pop" groceries, butcher shops, farmer's markets, roadside stands, etc. There are many lessons a child can learn while shopping for food.

When you take your child shopping with you, it has to be fun. If it's not, he will learn that the extra time it takes to get his own food is not worth the effort. He will learn from your attitude and from how you act while shopping.

I know ... grocery shopping can be a real bummer. The parking lot can be congested. The clerks sometimes seem to have taken a course in "How to Disappear When Customers Need Help." Many of the advertised sale items are out of stock. The line for rainchecks is half an hour long. The manager has decided to save energy by turning off the lights in the produce section, and it seems like you were dragging this same wobbly cart full of expensive, heavy groceries just yesterday!

I designed my markets and selected and trained my staff to make shopping a fun adventure, but the markets you shop in may not be so designed. That's no excuse. Remember, start with yourself. Examine your own attitude and go to work on it if you find yourself dreading market day.

Make the necessary changes. Find markets you enjoy. Shop at times when you—and the crowds—are more relaxed. If you've had a rough day, don't go to the market with your child if it's going to be stressful and unpleasant.

Remember that everything that goes on while your child is with you is a learning experience for him. If you silently go about your shopping, and only occasionally mumble to yourself or to him, the child will grow bored. He'll learn nothing positive about food.

Try making your child your shopping partner. Put him to work helping you select and put items into the cart. Always tell him what each item is, and relate it to his health the same way you did for the food. If he has never seen a spaghetti squash before it has been cooked and forked out of its skin, tell him what you are putting in the cart will be transformed into it's familiar, appetizing self soon.

This is a good time to connect foods with their nutritional value. As you put oranges in the cart, you can say, "Oranges help keep us from getting colds."

Allow your partner to choose some items, too. The safest area of the market to do this—if you're shopping in a store where all the food's not natural—is in the produce section. It's one thing for your child to be attracted to the bright colors of papayas or red cabbages. It's another problem entirely if the ten-foot high stack of Bonzo the Clown's Instant Artificial Brownies catches his eye. You can always find out how to serve a new fruit or vegetable, but what are you going to do with artificial brownies?

Whatever your partner chooses, put it in the cart. Then ask him why he chose it. Maybe he was attracted by the shape, color, or smell. Whatever his reason, here's your chance to strengthen his self-esteem. Don't say anything negative about his selection. Say something positive—even if you don't have the slightest idea what to do with it. If you've never used that particular fruit or vegetable before, admit it. But also say you're excited about this new adventure.

Then, find out how to prepare the item. Let your child in on the entire process. Keep the spirit cheerful and inquisitive. You and your partner are experimenting. So much of life is experimenting!

Encourage a free exchange of information on how everyone feels about this new food. If he doesn't enjoy it, affirm the positive: "Well, we can try to prepare it another way soon, if you like." Or ... "That was a good lesson. We learned that we don't especially like that food."

Make the experience a triumph for your child.

Grow Sprouts

Everyone responds to the magic of helping something grow, and one of the most effective gardening lessons you can do is to grow sprouts. Nothing you can say to a child can have a more inspiring effect than taking part in the wondrous bursting forth of the life force in seeds.

Sprouting is simple. Your child can do all of it himself, with a minimum of supervision. All you need to do is pour a tablespoon or two of seeds (alfalfa, sunflower, wheat grass, mung beans, soybeans, lentils, peas, garbanzos, rye, oats, corn, aduki, millet, or fenugreek) into a sprouting jar with an adequately screened lid. Rinse the seeds and drain excess water through the screen.

Cover the seeds with water and let them stand overnight—the first night only. Most seeds need to stand from six to twelve hours. Soybeans, however, need to soak longer—from twelve to twenty-four hours. Experiment with different lengths of soaking time until you find the time that works best for you.

Rinse again in the morning, and then at least three or four more times a day thereafter. They will begin to sprout within a day or two, and will be completely sprouted in three to six days, depending on the type of seed.

During and after the sprouting, talk to your child about the process. You can ask him to draw a picture, or a series of pictures, of the sprouting seeds as they appeared from bag to jar to salad. Ask him what he sees happening in the seeds and the sprouts.

Listen carefully to his ideas. Then try to express your explanation in the same terms he uses—by adding to his explanation, not subtracting from it. For example, he may say that the water goes into the seeds and pushes out the sprouts. That's a very direct way to view the process. Don't say, "No, that's not what happens. It happens like this ... ."

He will better learn the correct way if he can incorporate it into his own explanation rather than by having to dismantle his and replace it with yours. So if you can say something like, "Yes, that's right. The water goes into the seed and awakens very powerful forces of life that make the seed expand from the inside and push through the surface to grow into a sprout and then a plant," you are adding to his knowledge rather than challenging it with your own.

Carry the lesson a bit further. Say that by eating the sprout, we are allowing that powerful life force to work for *us* to make us healthy. Be careful to let the very young child understand that the life force of the sprout aids *his own growth*, but that the sprout itself does not keep growing inside him.

Bake Some Bread!

Baking bread involves all the senses. Your child can get real "hands on" stimulation from touching and measuring all the ingredients and kneading the dough. He can see and feel and smell all the different colors, textures, and aromas that combine to make the dough. Then he can witness the changes in texture and shape that the dough goes through on its way to becoming a loaf of bread. He can smell the exciting aroma of rising dough and baking bread.

To cap it all off, the taste of oven-fresh bread is the perfect conclusion to a lesson on where food comes from. He can even enjoy the crunch of the crust when he takes his first bite!

You can begin the bread baking experience by reading or telling the story of the Little Red Hen. Remember? The Little Red Hen had to grow the grain, harvest it, grind it, and finally bake the bread all by herself—with only her chicks to help her. Of course, she and her partners then had the satisfaction of eating the delicious bread all by themselves, too.

Before starting out, you can show your child photographs of a field of wheat and close-ups of wheat plants. You can even grow some wheat grass sprouts to show how a wheat plant starts out. You may even want to add some of these sprouts to your bread. If possible, you can purchase wheat berries and grind them into flour at home or at the store.

Any time you cook with your child, it's a good idea to explain all the steps before you start. You can even draw simple sketches to illustrate the adventure that's about to begin.

Before you get out the equipment and ingredients, decide what your child is going to do. Then, when you explain the process, highlight those responsibilities. Although it may mean more mess to clean up, don't try to prevent mistakes by limiting his role. The only valid limiting consideration should be his safety.

Allow him to do enough to proudly say, "This is my loaf of bread!" Knowing that his role was central rather than just helping will add to his satisfaction. Then, when you serve the loaf to the family, don't say, "Sammy *helped* me bake this loaf of bread." Say, with all truthfulness, "Sammy baked this loaf of bread today." You can do the same whenever you cook something with your child, and the accomplishment will nourish his sense of competence.

In the recipe section at the end of the book, you will find one of my favorite bread recipes: Auntie Sue's (Epstein) Whole Wheat Bread. I hope you and your family enjoy it as much as mine does.

Art

Encourage your child to draw pictures of whatever special activity you're about to do, or have already done. This gives him the opportunity to share his point of view with you. It also gives you the opportunity to see what's really on his mind.

You can expand the drawing into a language experience by asking him for a title for each picture. Or, you might suggest a title before he draws the picture. You can ask him to draw a series of pictures telling the story of each activity: "This is the way I looked when I was mixing the dough. This is the way I looked when I was petting the cow. This is the way I looked when I was putting the funny-looking vegetable in the shopping cart. This is the way Mommy looked when she was trying to cook the new vegetable."

You can also ask him about other sensory impressions while he's drawing, or afterwards. How did it feel to knead the dough? How did the baking bread smell? How did the bread taste? How did the farm smell? What sounds did you hear at the farm?

You can write his sense impressions on each drawing, so they can be read back to him later.

Ask your child to give a title for each picture—even the ones you've already titled. Write his title somewhere on the drawing, or on the back. His title is the word or group of words he relates to the experience. It may consist of several sentences. The picture and the title will give you important clues to his comprehension of the experience.

Don't jump to the conclusion that things he leaves out represent gaps in his knowledge. He may leave the fences out of the farm pictures. That doesn't necessarily mean he doesn't know they were there. It may mean he experienced the animals strongly despite the fences—a sign of independence and self-confidence.

Don't criticize the drawings. Use them to establish a dialogue with your child. He is telling you what he has seen and understood. Acknowledge that. Add gently to that vision if there are gaps, but don't dismantle it or overshadow it with your own.

This is your big chance to affirm his point of view. Do that by praising the drawings. Show that they awaken in you the same kind of excitement that the original experience did. Hang the pictures on the refrigerator door, or in some other highly-visible area. This will keep the lesson alive.

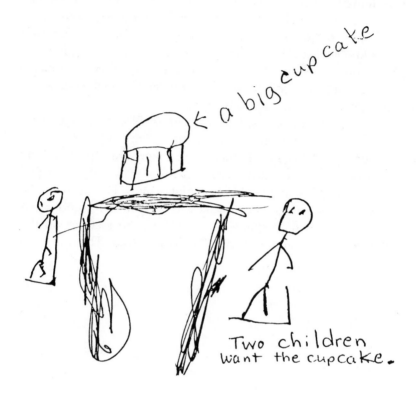

← a big cupcake

Two children want the cupcake.

Cup Cakes

Pour 2 spoons of milk in a pan. Then put 1 scoop of flour, 1 egg, and 2 cups of baking powder in. Mix this all up in a great big container, because we really got a lot of stuff in there.

Pour this in tiny rectangle things. Put it in a 70° oven for 1 hour.

Guy Lindsey

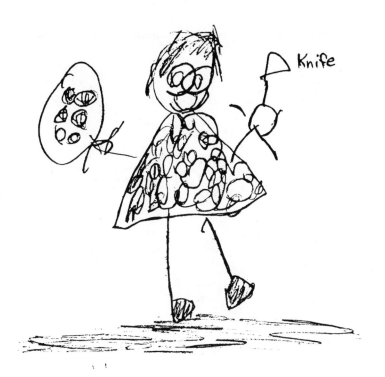

Plain Ole Salad

You need a middle sized bowl. Put in ½ head of chopped up lettuce, ½ celery, 5 chopped carrots, 10 big avocados, 6 cut up cucumbers, and some little bits of long onions.

For dressing, you mix up milk (what you drink for dinner) with white powder and ½ of a salt. Pour this over the salad and mix it up.

Serve this with spaghetti, rice and peas.

Kim Harvey

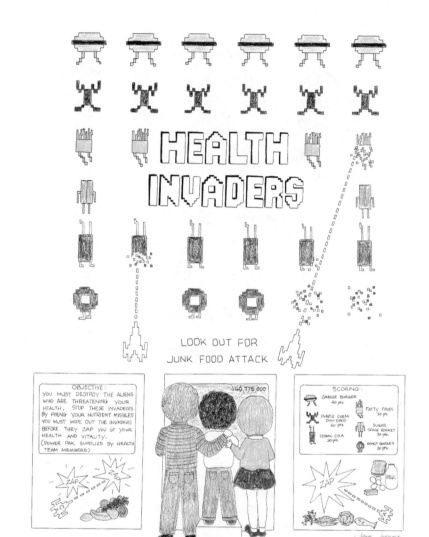

LOOK OUT FOR
JUNK FOOD ATTACK

Health Is A Beautiful Spaceship

7

Your nine year old will have more of the mental equipment to grasp some of the more complex relationships in nutrition. Unfortunately, she will also have had more time to be seduced into grasping some of the more perverse junk foods.

She's not going to innocently follow your lead the way a four year old will. She's developing the ability to understand complex chains of cause and effect. So you can get into deeper explanations of why some foods are good and others are not.

But she can get into deeper trouble by figuring out that she can spend her allowance on Greaseburgers and Fatty-fries after school.

She understands all too well the complex chain of cause and effect that says when she drops a quarter in the slot of the vending machine at school, she'll receive a hit of Purple Chemi-Doo-Dads.

She's growing in the ability to understand how parts fit together and make up a whole. You'll be able to more fully explain how specific nutrients (protein, carbohydrates, fats, vitamins, and minerals) combine in whole food.

But then, she'll also figure out that she can trade off parts of her lunch and not lose the whole meal.

She'll start thinking of her body as a collection of parts with individual functions, so you'll be able to talk to her about how specific nutrients help those parts do their thing. But because you've been taking such good care of her all her life, she'll have so much energy that it won't really hit home that she needs to take care of herself if she wants to hold on to that vitality.

You must still fit your message into her view of the world, but you'll have to work hard, because her view of the world begins and ends with herself. She's wrapped up pretty tight in the marvelous, growing creature that she is.

Her view of the world definitely does not include a working knowledge of biochemistry. At this stage of the game, she's more fascinated by the flashing colors of a video game than by images of chemicals choreographed into a complex, life-giving dance.

If visions of biochemicals working together won't yet fit into her head, perhaps images of people working in teams will. We can use the image of the team, with each member's contribution vital to its overall success, to help explain the Health Team of Nutrients working together to maintain her health and vitality.

The Health Team — Elements of Whole Food

Whole food maintains life and helps us do all that we want to do, and does it better than food that is not whole. Whole wheat bread is better than white bread. Brown rice is better than white rice. Honey is better than sugar.

That's the message we want our children to learn, and the Health Team can be used in a variety of ways to get it across. You can expand or shrink the scope of the team, depending on what you want to teach. For example, at its broadest, the Health Team can be pictured as all the elements of whole food—all the nutrients—working together to win the "game," our health and vitality. At the narrow end, you can have the Health Team made up of the eight essential amino acids that must be present for protein to be complete. Somewhere in between, you can envision a Health Team made up of the elements of a particular whole food. For example, whole wheat flour has all the team members it's supposed to have: germ, bran, B vitamins, etc. White flour, however, does not.

As with any team, if all the members aren't there when you need them, the entire effort suffers. If any member of the Health Team is not there to do its job, our body will not work as well as we would like it to.

When you're talking about Frozen Plastic Pies, Choco-sweets, and other junk food horrors, you can say that there are alien players in them, vandals who sneak in disguised as food but who have mayhem— not health—in their hearts.

Your child's world is abundant with teams. Choose a team she knows. If she's a member of an athletic team, use that sport for your example. The team you use should be dynamic. It should work when each member is in the right place at the right time, performing the right task. Each member's function should stand out as important to the total effort. Your child should be able to clearly picture what would happen if one or more members were taken away. Athletic teams, school bands and orchestras, and drama groups fit very well. A choir does not, because the absence of one or two members will not affect the music enough to impress a child. Children are fascinated by construction projects. If you and your child know enough about a construction team, you can use that model.

Ask your child about the goals of the model team. She should be able to talk about what the team wants to do and how it does it. If you use a baseball team, for example, she doesn't need to know the finer points of the game, but she should be able to tell you what will happen if the shortstop and second baseman are absent. You will want her to "get the picture" that the absence of one or more of the Health Team players will cause a similar disruption in the life-game being played in her body.

How To Use the Health Team Concept To Teach About Whole Food

When you are teaching your child about the elements of whole food, there are three basic messages you can communicate:

What purpose does the nutrient-team member serve?

What happens if the nutrient-team member is absent?

What foods bring this nutrient-team member into the body?

At the end of this book, Appendix A supplies information that will help you answer these questions for each member of the Health Team. This appendix is not intended to take the place of a more comprehensive, detailed study of nutrition. In the bibliography, I have recommended several books that will supply you with more information about the elements of whole food.

You can refer to this appendix and plug in the information about each nutrient-team member when talking about the Health Team with your child.

For example, the appendix entry for vitamin A reads:

Vitamin A

Vitamin A promotes the health of our eyes, skin, bones, teeth, mucous membranes, adrenal glands (which govern our response to stress) and the glands which secrete digestive juices. We need vitamin A to resist infection, grow, heal wounds, and adjust our eyesight to darkness. Food sources of vitamin A include yellow and orange vegetables, tomatoes, dark green leafy vegatables, liver, egg yolk, and dairy products.

To use this information, you might proceed as follows.
"Vitamin A is a very important member of the Heath Team. Some very important parts of our body depend on its being at its position, doing its job, every day. Our eyes, skin, bones, teeth, blood, and some very important glands inside our body all count on vitamin A.
"You know what would happen if a catcher in a baseball game weren't at her position, don't you? Every time the pitcher threw the ball, there would be no one there to catch it if the batter didn't hit it! Think of how hard it would be for the team to play the game.
"It's the very same thing with Vitamin A. If vitamin A isn't there to do its job, our body will not work as well as we would like it to. Our eyes may not see well because vitamin A isn't there to do its job. We may find ourselves getting tired more easily when we're playing or working (since vitamin A supports the blood, adrenal glands, and digestion). We may get colds and flu more often, and our cuts and bruises may not heal as quickly as before.
"Vitamin A is so important that children who don't get enough of it for very long periods of time sometimes don't grow as big and strong as they could if they got what their body needed.
"But we won't allow vitamin A to be absent from our diet. We know how to bring this player to our Health Team. Every time we eat liver, eggs, milk, cheese, yogurt, or vegetables such as spinach, squash, carrots, and tomatoes, we're bringing in some vitamin A to our Health Team. Isn't it wonderful that we can do that?"
Of course, the body's Health Team has many more players than an athletic team, and the "game" is more complex. It may take a child a very long time to absorb a truly comprehensive understanding of every nutrient's importance and food sources. This knowledge can be one of

your long-range goals. A more immediately attainable goal can be to increase her appreciation of whole, natural food.

I have found that children will hold on to one or two specific purposes and symptoms that capture their imagination, and then link these with a favorite food that happens to be among the sources for that nutrient. For example, they may ask for oranges or orange juice because they want to make sure there's enough vitamin C on their team—so they won't catch cold, or so their cuts and scrapes will heal faster.

That is the open door you are looking for. The best information you can carry through it is that whole, natural foods will keep that team member—and all the others—in the game.

Taking an Older Child to a Farm

You can discuss the farm trip in more sophisticated terms with an older child, but the fundamental lesson is the same: food comes from living things. Try talking about how food was produced many years ago compared to how it is produced today. Discuss how this has affected food.

Taking the Older Child Shopping

Once your child understands the Health Team concept, you can begin to teach her to read labels. She now has a very effective tool for making selections. She knows she has to gather certain essential players and avoid the vandals. She has a picture in her mind of the importance of whole food.

Naturally, she doesn't yet have a working knowledge of all ingredients. That comes with time and your help. As you shop, read the labels with her. Identify one ingredient at a time as either a good player or a vandal.

For example: "Whole wheat flour. That's a very good player .... Sodium nitrite—uh oh! That's an alien player—a vandal. We don't want that on our team." Demonstrate by the tone of your voice and your expression that the player is either welcome or to be avoided.

After a few trips, your child may be able to tell you whether an ingredient is a good player or a vandal. As you read the ingredients, ask her, "Do you want this player on your team?"

Of course, if you have already learned where all the good foods are in your market, you will have to pick up and read the labels on some foods you know you don't want—for academic purposes. Just be careful not to be too melodramatic when you read the label on the Purple Chemi-Doo-Dads and the Choco-sweets.

If your child is old enough to read labels by herself, let her go on a treasure hunt to find good food. Go over her choices with her. If she makes an error and brings back a vandal food, don't make a big deal out of it. Simply point out the vandal and tell her to try again.

Eventually, your child can be a full partner in your shopping excursions. But even more important than that, she will have learned how to choose a winning team when she selects food for herself.

Growing Sprouts

A sprout is actually a Health Team "farm." As the life forces go to work, the nutrients start to multiply. After a day or two, the concentrations of vitamins are many times higher than in either the seed or the mature plant. When you talk about sprouting with an older child, make it clear that a sprout is about as far as you can get from Sugar Rockets and Doughnut Doodles.

Baking Bread

Follow the same steps as outlined for younger children in Chapter 6, but allow your older child to assume more responsibility. Ask him to suggest ways to "customize" the recipe by adding raisins, nuts, different blends of flours, etc.

Art

You can follow the same plan for artwork as outlined in the section for young children in Chapter 6, except that with older children you can use a wider variety of materials and media. Allow your child to choose from among crayons, pen and ink, charcoal, pastels, water-colors, chalk, poster paints, and modeling clay. Even Purple Chemi-Doo-Dads may at last have some useful purpose—as part of a junk food collage!

Teaching Nutrition to Teenagers

I'm sure you know by now that a teenager tends to be more in-dependent than a younger child. You may need to work hard to reach the teen on her own terms, but once you do go all the way and start fit-ting bits of knowledge into her world, watch out! Your teen will re-spond in ways that the younger child cannot.

Teenagers are beginning to get a real feel for the *power* of knowledge. They love to use their new reasoning tools to win arguments, so be sure you have your facts straight. Even then, be careful to approach the burgeoning intellect in a friendly, sharing way. Teens may love to learn, but they can also hate to be taught.

Teens have a more sophisticated spectrum of interests. They are very sensitive to any intrusion on their right to decide what is relevant to their lives. You may have to come in the back door and bring your nutrition lessons along in a box labeled "politics," "economics," "history," or some other "relevant" interest.

Teens care what their friends think. They derive a lot of their self-esteem from their status among their peers. What determines their status? More than any other factors: their appearance and their perform-ance in sports, schoolwork, and extracurricular activities.

An open door! You can use you teen's interest in appearance and performance to get through her "relevance barriers." What could be more relevant than information that could keep her skin clear and her hair shining?

Before you rush up to your teenager with statements such as "Whole wheat bread and yogurt and wheat germ and vitamins will turn you into a movie star and an athlete all at once!"—make sure your own knowledge of the relationships between nutrition and appearance and performance is sophisticated enough to answer the questions that will eventually come up. For a start, the Health Team image can be used to establish that food does affect performance and appearance, but you'll need to do additional research to carry the relationships further into specific problem areas.

You may also gain entry into your teen's world by means of scholastic interests. For example, if she favors political science or economics, you can talk about natural foods in terms of the economic laws of supply and demand. It is now profitable for the food industry to continue to sell manufactured food, but we have the power to eradicate Choco-sweets and Sugar Rockets and Doughnut Doodles and Frosted Fruit Barrels virtually overnight. All we have to do is stop buying them. Production follows demand. Demand follows education.

If your teen is interested in ecology, start with a discussion of how certain aspects of modern food technology disrupt the balance of nature. Move from there to how manufactured food disrupts the balance of nature within our own bodies.

As children grow older, their naturally strong curiosity becomes matched with an increasingly powerful intellectual machinery for exploring, observing, experimenting, and reasoning. Your teenager has the intellectual equipment to find out more about nutrition than *you* know.

Think of this as an advantage rather than a threat. Once you manage to ignite your teen's curiosity, all you'll really have to do is point her in the direction of books, lectures, experiments, courses, people to talk to, and other avenues of research.

Then ... get out of the way! Or, better still, let your own curiosity shine, too. There's no reason why you can't do just as much research as your teenager!

Special Activities

Your teen may not be as cooperative as a younger child in taking on special activities. While a younger child will jump at the chance to visit a farm—for the pure fun of it!—a teen may balk. Perhaps it's also true that you can't really ask a teenager to draw a picture of a farm as part of a lesson, either.

Nevertheless, there are other approaches you can take to get your teen to cooperate, after a fashion. First, you can combine two or more activities at once. Second, you can ask her to do you a favor.

For example, combine the farm visit with a shopping trip for farm-fresh produce, meat, milk, or eggs—like Sue Epstein did in Germany. Combine the farm visit with art, by asking your teen to use her special artisitic talents to memorialize the visit. You can even combine bread baking and art by asking her to shape the loaves into people, animals ... whatever!

Get the idea?

Children of all ages enjoy helping their parents—most of the time— so don't be afraid to ask your teenager to do you a favor and please help out with the shopping. Of course, she'll have to shop by your standards. In order to do that, she'll have to learn your standards, which means learning to read labels.

You can use the "please do me a favor" approach to get your teen to grow some sprouts for salads or lunches, and she ought to be more than happy to help you bake bread. Remember the Little Red Hen?

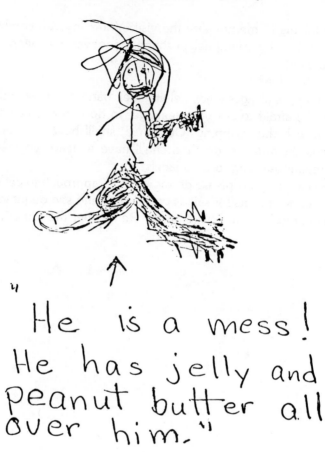

⁴
"He is a mess!
He has jelly and
peanut butter all
over him."

A Soft Sandwich

Get out the bread and 5¢ worth of peanut butter and a $1.30 worth of strawberry jelly. Put this together.

If this sticks in your mouth, take a finger and push it off.

Dennis Sanford

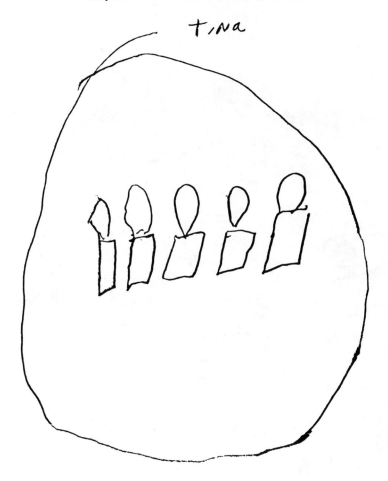

Vanilla Cake

You need 1 cup of sugar, 2 cups of vanilla, 1 cup of flour and 2 eggs. Mix it all up. Put it in the oven. (But our oven doesn't work, so we better put it in a pancake griddle and cook it that way.) It will look like a giant pancake when it is cooked.
Put frosting and 5 candles on it.

Tina Rudy

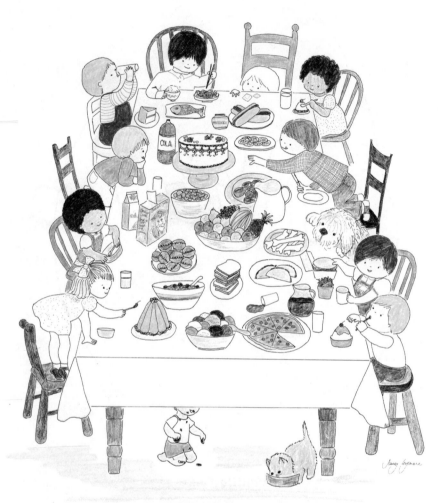

Kids Eat the Darnedest Things

8

We want to change our children's eating habits. We want to replace their unhealthy patterns with new, natural, healthy ones. But where did these unhealthy patterns come from?

What better place to start our search than the supermarket, where all the junk comes from in the first place—right?

There's a young mother going in now. Let's follow her. She looks reasonably intelligent, healthy, and sincere. Better still, she doesn't have any children with her, so we know she is not going to be influenced by a child demanding Choco-sweets and Sugar-Bunnies.

Good. The first thing she puts in her shopping cart is chicken. Ah! Whole wheat bread. This woman knows her nutrition!

Uh-oh. She's headed for the canned food section at a pretty good clip. She's noticed that there's a sale on sugar-packed canned peaches, pears, and fruit cocktail, and she's loading cans into her cart by the case!

Now she's heading for the cereal section—no doubt to pick up some wheat germ and granola and whole grain breakfast cereals?

Nope. Three family-size boxes of Sugar Wheats.

Oh dear ... she's picking up speed as she heads for the dessert area. Now she's loading boxes of sweetened gelatin dessert into her cart! On no! She's heading for the cake mixes ... slowing down ... reaching for ... three boxes of cake mix! ... And three cans of frosting mix! Arrrrgh!

I suppose we might as well follow her the rest of the way. Oh good—she's picking up some salad greens ... some fresh fruit ... some frozen orange juice ... and—uggh!—diet soda. Chocolate milk! Frozen vegetables with sugary sauces!

She's heading for the checkouts. Thank goodness she's done. Oops—spoke too soon. She's loading up with chocolate bars ... .

We've followed this woman through the supermarket for two reasons. First, because she's answered our original question for us. How do our children develop unhealthy eating habits? They do it by eating the unhealthy foods we purchase for them. The junk food habit begins with what happens on those shopping trips—whether there's a screaming demanding child along or not. We parents put the food into the shopping cart, for better or worse.

The second reason I followed this woman through the market is because ... she is—or *was*—Sandy Gooch, back in the mid-seventies. The above is a perfect description of my typical shopping trip, before I learned—the hard way—about the health value and importance of natural foods.

The chocolate bars and the diet soda were all for me. And as for the gelatin and canned fruit ... well, *nothing* was better on our Sugar Wheats than canned fruit. Ugh! Can you believe it? Among our friends I was literally *known* for my gelatin molds. I would make them with three different layers—each layer a different color. Canned mandarin oranges on the first layer, fruit cocktail on the second, and canned peaches on the third.

Why do we do it?

We do it for a lot of reasons, but most often because it's just the easiest thing—the path of least resistance. Or maybe we just don't know any better. We're not totally aware of what the food is doing to us, so we just buy what's advertised.

Children learn to eat the darnedest things because we teach them to do it. We *parents* succumb to the pressures of the advertisers and the supermarket layout and design, and the need to find something to eat—and find it *fast*.

After all, children get most of their food—and *all* their first food—from us. I've talked to many parents who have told me that their children have never had any junk—*and they don't miss it.*

I've also heard from too many parents who've come into the store for the first time admitting that their children came home and *insisted* they buy natural food after participating in one of the tours of Mrs. Gooch's Markets I conduct for schoolchildren. One mother came in and told me her daughter came home from the tour very excited about natural foods—and proceeded to convert the entire family. Another mother told me her daughter absolutely *refused* to eat the sugary cereal she gave her for breakfast, "because it's not natural!"

I am sharing these stories in hopes of taking some of the pressure off the children. They don't create their own unhealthy eating habits. We do it for them. The children aren't the conservative ones. They're not the ones in the family who will be most resistant to changes. We adults are.

Children *learn* to like what we give them. They get used to it first. Then, when they see that it pleases us when they eat what we give them, they connect the food with the love and acceptance they get from us. Children—and adults—may have a sweet tooth for candy and other confections, but our most powerful sweet tooth is for *love*.

Unfortunately, in this day and age, we seem to feel that the best way to show love is by satisfying someone's sweet tooth! On Valentine's Day, we show our love with a big box of chocolates. Easter baskets overflow with candy eggs and chocolate bunnies. "Nothing says 'lovin' like something in the oven," the commercial croons, and more often than not, the something that's in the oven is a sugary cake mix loaded with preservatives and other artificial chemicals.

If Johnnie gets restless and starts fidgeting in the supermarket, Mom says, "Be a good boy and I'll buy you a chocolate bar at the checkout on the way out." Those convenient shelves full of candy aren't there by accident, you know.

Do you think it's really the hamburger or the fried chicken that Susie or Billy wants when they see the commercial for the fast food restaurant? No ... it's the experience of going somewhere accepted— somewhere validated by a TV commercial—with people you love.

Have you ever stopped to think of all the feelings we communicate by means of food? We use food to express love, forgiveness, acceptance, happiness, congratulations, condolences, passion, celebration ... the list goes on and on.

The point is that when you set out to change the unhealthy eating habits of your children and family, you are, in effect, announcing: "*We are now going to start showing love around here in a new way.*" Does this mean you're going to stop using food to communicate love, acceptance, and other feelings? No. That would be very difficult, if not impossible. The purpose of this book is not to get you to stop showing love with food, but to help you start showing love with *good food*.

As a matter of fact, that might not be such a bad way to begin—by actually announcing to your child, and the rest of the family, that "From now on, we are going to show love around here in a new way—with good, healthy, natural food."

Isn't It Easier To Be Sneaky About It?

A lot of homemakers come to me and wonder out loud whether they—and their families—wouldn't be better off if they carried out their natural foods revolution on the sly. You know what I mean—by adding wheat germ, liver, bran, and a host of other healthy ingredients to the mostly unhealthy junk they're accustomed to eating. (Can you appreciate the absurdity of adding four tablespoons of wheat germ to a chocolate cake mix loaded with artificial chemicals and sugar—and expecting the wheat germ to make it good for you?)

I know this method has "worked" for some people. There's no question that, on a purely nutritional basis, the family that's having wheat germ and other natural food supplements added to its food on the sly is better off than the family that's eating totally devitalized food, but this method is not for me.

If you go this route and sneak natural goodies into your family's diet, you're not teaching them anything. They're not going to learn that natural foods are better, and they're certainly not going to learn how to make healthy food choices for themselves. You won't always be there to tamper with their food supply, either.

Also, I *know* there's an energy flow connected with food. If there weren't, why would we use food to communicate so many powerful feelings? It seems to me that if we misrepresent the food we give to others, if we give them something and they aren't aware of what we're giving them, the energy that flows between us is going to be affected in some negative way. After all, worrying about whether they'll find out what you're giving them—and worrying because you're not telling the truth about the food—are negative feelings, and these negative feelings are going to be imparted into the food.

"OK, Sandy, you've talked me out of being sneaky. You've told me to go out and announce to the whole family that we're going to dump the junk and devote ourselves to good food. They're all looking at me ... a little scared ... wondering whether I've gone off my rocker or something ... wondering if this means they're going to have to give up their hamburgers and their spaghetti and meatballs and their hot dogs and their cookies and pies ... but ... *Sandy, what do I do next?*"

The first thing you do is let them know that you're going to be *adding* to their lives—not subtracting.

Next, let them know you're going to be supportive of them and not try to totally overhaul *every* one of those habits that took so long to develop. In other words, you're not going to bury them with a barrage of bean sprouts and wheat germ. Let them know that, for the most part, they will still be able to enjoy their favorite foods—only now they'll be natural. Ask them for their support and help, and ...

Then ... get to work! Slowly begin, with dedication and patience, to change their patterns of eating.

"But, Sandy, how can we go slowly if we have a pantry full of junk food and the gang is waiting for their hamburgers and Fatty-fries?"

I'm asked this question a lot. What you're really asking is how can I begin slowly and yet not compromise what I know to be the best way to feed my children?

Some people prefer to go cold turkey—to just go on a raiding rampage through the pantry and dump all the junk in the trash. I was *forced* to go that route. My family accepted the fact that I had to go on a totally natural foods diet *immediately*—or stay very ill. So everyone rolled with the punches, and watched the junk disappear virtually overnight.

Most people don't change that quickly. Chances are, your own education in natural foods will be a gradual process. You *will* be able to educate your children slowly and patiently, as you, yourself, learn about natural foods.

You have a real job to do. As close as you might be to your children, they—and the rest of your family—are not inside your head. They won't know what's going on in there unless you share it with them, so don't be afraid to sit down and really tell them what's going on with you and all these natural foods. Your main job is to convince them that you're *adding* to their lives, not taking away.

You have to *plan your approach*. You have to figure out for yourself what "gradual" means to you. Does it mean that you will plan to have the diet totally natural within three months, six months, a year?

How are you going to start changes? Are you going to bring in fresh fruits and vegetables, then natural meats, then whole grains? Or, are you going to approach it on a meal-by-meal basis: first, throw out the sugary breakfast cereals, then tackle lunch, then supper?

Make Every Shopping Trip Count

Most people shop at least once a week. Once your consciousness about nutrition and natural foods has reached a certain level and you know that one item is better than another, are you going to purchase the item that you *know* isn't as good? Of course not. You will want to make every shopping trip as perfect as it can be.

Here's a wonderful place to enlist your children's help. As you teach them more and more about nutrition, you can let them participate in your shopping trips by helping you read the labels on the food you buy.

The important thing is not how fast or how perfect or how complete your natural foods revolution is in the beginning. What's important is that you set out from the very first to maintain an environment for honesty and flexibility.

Affirm the Positive

The best way to get a child—or an adult, for that matter—to accept a change and adapt to a new situation is to express it in positive terms. Allow them to see the change as an improvement rather than as a problem or a deterioration. Natural foods is a new *adventure* you're embarking on, not a trial to endure. *This is going to be fun!*

Take the approach that this is going to be better all around—and don't be afraid to explain why. The "teaching chapters" are in this book to help you do just that—teach your children about natural foods.

Please don't make the change to natural foods into some kind of archaic, pseudo-religious sacrifice: "This is good for us ... and even if it tastes terrible, we're going to do it!" Put away the hairshirts.

Instead, put your child's attention on good things that are going to come out of this new adventure. Natural foods taste better. They look better. And they *are* better, nutritionally.

Think about the things that went into your own decision to switch to natural foods—and share them with your children and the rest of your family. Put your child's attention on the positive things that are going to happen because of these changes. Tell him the food will make him healthier—he'll feel better, look better, work better, and play better. The teaching chapters will tell you how to do this most efficiently for your child's age level.

Substitution is the Key

The best way to convince your children that natural foods are really OK is to demonstrate that they're not going to have to give up their favorite foods—at least, not all of them. The health food industry has come a long way in the last decade or so. Now, you can find natural whole grain hot dog and hamburger buns, natural hot dogs and hamburgers and natural mustard, mayonnaise, relish, and catsup to adorn them. You can find whole grain pasta ... whole grain instant cereals ... natural soda pops sweetened with honey, cookies, and cakes. When you come right down to it, you can find natural versions of everything from pizza to ice cream.

There's no reason your children should give up their All-American diet while you're switching to natural foods. Let them know they're going to have the same favorite foods as before—only now they'll be better.

Some Things Are Going To Have To Go

Of course, this is not to discourage you from changing their diet in more fundamental ways. Maybe you *want* to get the hamburgers and hot dogs out of their diet. That decision is yours to make. But the same rule applies: substitute something you know they'll love for the item you are, in effect, taking away.

Even if you're not making such drastic, fundamental changes in your child's diet, it's true that some things are going to have to go. You can't duplicate *every* food with a natural, healthy version. Some foods—like sugary breakfast cereals, for example—don't lend themselves to natural duplication. Plastic, totally worthless junk food will simply have to disappear.

You can still substitute natural goodies for the garbage you're getting rid of, and I've included several recipes in Appendix B to help you do just that. You're still going to have a real teaching job ahead of you to help your child get over the bumps of not having his favorite candy bar or candy cereal for breakfast. If you're open and honest and sharing, I have found that children really do understand reasons.

Love is on Your Side

I started this chapter by saying that our children's hunger for junk food originates with us, their parents. We can use this to our advantage in helping our children break these unhealthy eating patterns that we created.

One of the reasons our children learned to love junk is because it came along with our love for them. We let them lick the bowl after we made that sugary cake. We bought them the candy bar when they were good. We went to all the trouble to make that gigantic batch of cookies for their birthday party.

Now, we can get that same wonderful feeling of love to work its magic on our natural foods revolution. We can still let the child lick the bowl—only now the cake will be a honey, whole wheat carrot cake. He can still get a "candy bar"—only now it will be a sugarless carob-raisin-date bar. And there will still be gigantic batches of cookies. Only now, they'll be whole grain oatmeal cookies, made with honey and other natural ingredients.

Love can help you over the rough spots. When you want your child to *try* a new, wonderful natural food, you can simply say, "Please try this _____ that Mommy (or Daddy) made *just for you.*"

Freedom Works Wonders

As you progress and change your child's eating habits, you will eventually be asking, and relying on, him to make choices for himself. That's a new responsibility in his life. And, if you remember our six working principles, with every responsibility comes freedom. Whenever you give your child a responsibility, also give him a choice. If you want him to help cook dinner, allow him to choose what he'll be doing from a number of options. Allow him to choose part of the menu, too.

Give him the freedom to choose as often as possible. This will help him get used to exercising the real responsibility that comes with freedom. He'll learn to own up to his decisions and their consequences.

You don't want your child to be intimidated by freedom and life's possiblities, do you? I've read that when certain animals that have been born and raised in zoos are set free in wild game preserves—where they have virtually unlimited freedom of movement—they often pace back and forth in an area no larger than their former cages! I'm sure we've all known people who suffered from this same self-limiting attitude. They've never learned how to deal with freedom.

Likewise, it's not always easy for us to "let go" and watch a child exercise freedom, especially when the child is older and the stakes are higher. That's why it's necessary to make freedom part of your every-day relationship with your child—in particular, part of every step in your change to a better, healthier, more natural diet.

As you progress, allow him to make more and more decisions. For example, when you're ordering a meal at a restaurant, let him choose his own meal. Sounds simple enough, but how many times have you heard yourself say, "But you had that once before and didn't like it!" Or, "Not that! You'll make a mess on your clothes!"

You *can* let your child choose what he wants—and then support that choice. Maybe he will choose a certain dish and then discover that it's not as good as he thought it would be. *So what?* Hasn't that ever happened to you?

What are you going to do about it if it does happen? Are you going to shout (or whisper), "I told you you wouldn't like it! I'll never let you choose again!" Or are you going to make yourself human and vulnerable to him, by saying: "I guess you don't like it as much as you thought you would. Well, that's OK. Sometimes I make the wrong decision, too. Once I ordered something I thought I would absolutely love, and it almost made me sick!" Isn't that better?

Freedom can work wonders when it's given the chance. A few years ago, a husband and wife who had suddenly become very strict vegetarians came to me with a problem they were having with their nine year old son. Their son did not appear to be quite as enthusiastic about vegetarianism as they were—to put it mildly.

"We don't know what to do," they said. "We give him marvelous lunches to take to school, and then we find out that he's trading them for jam sandwiches and hot dogs. And lately, we've been finding candy wrappers under his mattress!"

The parents always followed up these discoveries with lectures, scoldings, and further restrictions. The poor parents were desperate. Neither had the slightest idea what to do next.

I could tell this situation called for drastic measures. The following is what I told them.

"It's sometimes very difficult for a child to accept a concept that we embrace. You have to give him time and freedom to make the choices himself. Why don't you try—just as an experiment—allowing your son to have one or maybe two days a week when he can eat *anything he wants*, and offer to get it for him. Take him anywhere he wants to go—even if it's a fast food restaurant or a candy store.

"If he wants to stuff himself full of junk, let him do it. Allow him that freedom. Let him know that you care about him enough to let him begin to make his own decisions. In the meantime, of course, he will cooperate with your regular diet. That's part of the deal, but don't make a big thing out of it. Just make it your way of life. No lectures. OK?"

My friends were a bit stunned by my suggestion, but they were so desperate that they said they would try anything. So they gave it a try.

They came back about two months later and said, "Sandy, it worked like a charm. When Saturday comes around, we say, 'OK, today's your day to choose. What do you want to eat?'

"The first two or three Saturdays were nightmares of junk food. But now, when Saturday rolls around, he just says, 'Well ... I don't really want to do that today. Maybe I'll just skip this week.'

"Sandy, he's still skipping weeks—after all these weeks!"

This child kept on "skipping weeks" because he began to feel that he was not being pressured anymore, that he had more freedom, and that *he* could make the choices. Maybe he really never wanted to do things like trade his lunch or sneak candy bars into his room. Maybe he did these things partly to protest his parents' rigidity and partly out of resentment—inner rage that they were not allowing him enough of the freedom and responsibility he knew he was ready to handle.

His rebellion was a statement that *he was an individual*. As soon as his father and mother acknowledged that—with action as well as words—there was no longer any need to rebel. He could participate in his family's way of life as a free, responsible member of the family.

My friends' situation involved drastic tensions and restrictions, so it also required a drastic dose of freedom. In extreme circumstances, we sometimes need extreme solutions—solutions we would not normally consider. For example, surgery is a drastic step for anyone to take. We would not want to have surgery unless it were the only choice available. We would also prefer not to have to expose our children to junk food, but in this case, such an extreme course was necessary.

My aim in this book is to help you avoid the kind of drastic solution my vegetarian friends had to employ. If you acknowledge and protect your child's freedom right from the start, you will succeed.

Special Activities

Art

Have your child make a menu of his favorite foods—as if he were offering them in a restaurant of his own. He can be as artistic as he pleases in decorating the menu. He may want to make several menus, since he probably has several favorites that may lend themselves to different kinds of restaurants. Or, he may just want to make a variety of menus. Give his art free reign.

Shopping

Take your child shopping on a treasure hunt for natural versions of his favorite foods. Let him help you find them, or the ingredients to make them naturally.

Cooking

Prepare these favorite foods along with him. In Appendix B, you will find several recipes of children's favorites. One of those recipes, the one for pumpkin bread, was devised by a young boy named Matt—a former student of mine—who converted his favorite dessert recipe himself. His mother converted another favorite recipe, which also appears. In this same appendix, you will find conversion tables and a substitution guide for making natural versions of children's favorite foods.

Have fun!

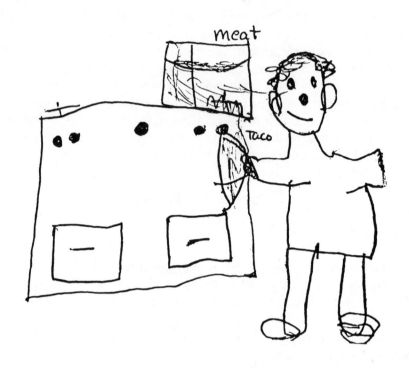

Tacos

Put a round thing in the frying pan with no grease. After it is cooked you gotta cook hamburger in a big pan, 'cuz it's for a lot of people. Mash up cheese and put it all over the meat. Put the meat on the round thing. Then start eating *fast!*

I hate hot sauce, so don't serve any of that.

Scott Lambright

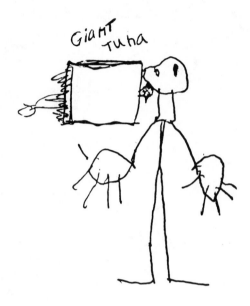

Tuna Sandwich

You take 3 cups of mayonnaise. Put in 3 cups of relish, and 3 cups of tuna. Stir it up. Put all this on 1 slice of bread—put the other slice on top.

This sandwich will be 12 inches high. You need a big mouth!

Danny Alling

But my Friends Eat Junk all the time!

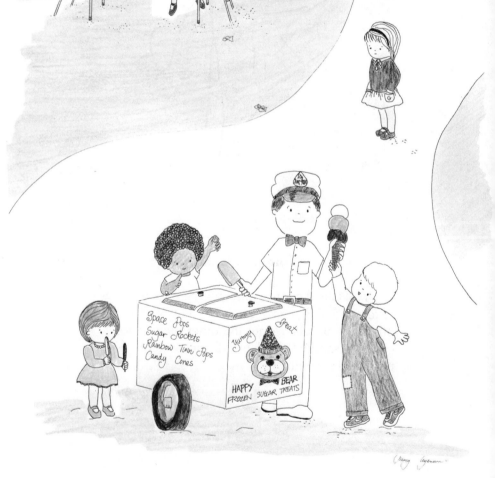

9

Sooner or later, your little girl is going to venture out into the cold, cruel neighborhood ... where the local ragamuffins lurk, ready to tempt her with Purple Chemi-Doo-Dads.

Maybe they'll lure your innocent child home—where their parents are, right this moment, loading the microwave with Friendly Frozen Fatty Fries to offer your unsuspecting child.

Or maybe your little girl will burst in the door one day with little Jackie from down the street not far behind, carrying a bag of Raunchy Rockets Snack Chips, or some similar nutritional disaster. And your child will say, "Look at what Jackie gets to eat at her house! Can we buy these, huh?"

Or ... "Jackie eats these, and she says they're great. She wants me to have some, too! Can I? Huh?"

Or ... even worse ... the children won't come to your house, but the phone will ring and it'll be Jackie's mom, who'll say: "We're having a snack of Friendly Frozen Fatty Fries and Captain Cool Junk Juice, and your daughter said she'd have to ask you first. I just thought I'd call and let you know. It's OK with you, isn't it?"

You have two options in dealing with situations like this. Your first option is to take a look at this chapter and try some of my suggestions for dealing with peer pressure. Your second option is to pack up the family and move to the Yukon territory, or some other wilderness area where you won't have to worry about neighbors and their children tempting your child away from the natural foods diet you've worked so hard to maintain.

If Option #1 doesn't do the trick, you can always resort to Option #2 ... .

Put Peer Pressure To Work
for You and Your Child

Peer pressure can work both ways. The challenge is to make it work *for* you and your child rather than against you. Once you understand how peer pressure works, it's not that difficult to use it to your own advantage.

Peer pressure works by appealing to our basic need to be accepted. As I said at the beginning of Chapter 3, we ideally learn to accept ourselves, so that self-love and validation come from within us.

Nevertheless, in addition to self-acceptance, we all need some measure of acceptance from the people around us. It's a very rare person who has so much self-acceptance and self-love that he doesn't need a slap on the back and an invitation to join the party every now and then.

Our children are no different. They want their peers to accept them, slap them on the back, and invite them to join in the fun. It's just coincidental that the "fun" sometimes happens to include Purple Chemi-Doo-Dads. Being included in the group supplies the real nourishment for the child's self-esteem. We parents can try to nourish our child's self-esteem in such a way as to do two things: make her better able to deal with peer pressure, and make *her* the *leader* from whom the other children receive peer pressure and influence.

The very first thing you can do is talk to your child about her feelings. Try to find out whether she is aware of how much better off she is, physically and emotionally, on a diet of natural foods. Again, this is basically an educational task. I feel that if a child is aware of how good she feels, her self-esteem will follow closely behind.

How has your switch to natural foods demonstrably affected your child's health? Look again at the reasons you decided to switch to natural foods in the first place. Use the educational tools in the earlier chapters to establish the connection between your child's health, her strength and vigor, and the natural foods diet. Once she knows that her body and mind function better on natural foods, she will have a source of nourishment for her self-esteem. Once she realizes that she feels better and looks better, her self-esteem will be ready for the peer pressure that tries to pull her away from natural foods. She'll also be better prepared to become the *leader* of her friends, so that they will want to follow in *her* dietary footsteps.

Encourage Your Child To Be the Leader

It's one thing to be able to make your child understand why your family is on a natural foods diet. It's another to explain why *everybody* isn't eating natural foods—especially Jackie down the street, who does seem to be having a lot of fun with those Friendly Frozen Fatty Fries.

You can deal with issues like this by saying: "Yes, Jackie does have Fatty Fries, and white bread, and candy bars, and (whatever else it happens to be) ... I have a feeling that Jackie and her parents don't know as much about nutrition as we do. If they did, they would know that white bread doesn't have all the vitamins and minerals and fiber that whole wheat bread does. They would also know that Fatty Fries and diet soda and baloney sandwiches have a lot of artificial chemicals added to them.

"Aren't we lucky that we are helping our bodies to grow in a healthy way by eating natural foods and not eating things like that? I feel sorry that Jackie and her family don't have the opportunity to do that right now. Maybe we can help them learn more about nutrition."

While you're encouraging your child to be the leader, also caution her against coming on too strong with her friends. There are many times when a child enjoys being a little different—as long as she isn't too weird. This is one area where she can stand out and be the "expert in the field," but we certainly don't want her running off to Jackie's house with fire in her eyes to preach the gospel of natural foods and condemn the junk food-eating "sinners" to bad health.

Converting the neighborhood can come later. Right now, what we want is for your daughter to be able to say and do the right thing when peer pressure tempts her with junk food.

What is the "right thing"? Well, something like, "No, I can't eat that because people who eat that stuff are going to die" may certainly get the job done, but it will probably close some doors on your child in the neighborhood. She's not going to win any votes for *leader* with campaign speeches like that! A simple, "No, thank you", will do the trick in most cases.

When Jackie or Jackie's mom press a little harder, your child can say, "No, *I don't really care for* Purple Chemi-Doo-Dads and Friendly Frozen Fatty Fries, thank you." Later in this chapter, we'll get into what to do when the pressure is even greater—when it's really important to Jackie and her mom that your daughter share their junk food.

Make Your House the Center

Your daughter's campaign for "leader" is going to be won or lost at your house—not the neighbors'. Two vitally important elements of that campaign are going to be carried out at your house. The first one, we've already talked about—the education of your child. The second depends a lot on you. The best way for your child to share her feelings about how good natural food can be is to actually share natural food with her friends.

There are several ways you can do this. Your first goal is to demonstrate to your child's friends that natural food isn't so bad after all and that, in fact, it can be far more delicious than the junk food they get elsewhere. You can accomplish this by having the children over for snacks, for breakfast, lunch, or dinner.

When my daughter, Kristin, was younger, I made my home the snack center of the neighborhood. The children would always want to come to my house because I made it fun for them. I absolutely adored having them there, so we would have a lot of fun baking things. Of course, I didn't mind the flour all over the floor, either.

You may not want to go that far, but you can still prepare some wholesome snacks to serve the children when they drop over with your daughter. *Show* Jackie and her other friends that apple juice and whole wheat peanut butter brownies can be loads better than Fatty Fries and Captain Cool Junk Juice!

Don't do a heavy number talking about how this or that natural food is *better for them* than whatever it is they may be getting at home. You want to appeal to their curiosity, their taste buds, their sense of adventure, and to their desire for fun.

Of course, Jackie is likely to ask you *why* you eat this "stuff" instead of Fatty Fries. In that event, you can say, "Because we like it better. Don't you think it tastes good?"

Once Jackie acknowledges that the natural food tastes good, the door is open for some information about the health benefits of natural food. That information may be better received, however, if it comes from your child rather than from you. Children sometimes have inborn defenses against adults telling them about anything that is good for them. If your daughter lets them know that this "natural stuff" not only tastes great but also helps her feel better, the information is more likely to find an open door.

Another way for your child to share her natural foods experience with her friends is for you to pack extra snacks and goodies in her lunch. Kristin's sack lunch would often bulge with extra sunflower seeds or natural munchies of one sort or another.

Children really do respond when you incorporate them into the whole scheme of things, and they understand that natural foods can be a plus in their lives rather than a minus. To do that, you can take the same tack that we talked about in the previous chapter. Let them know that eating natural foods doesn't mean giving up their All-American Favorites.

Just recently, Kristin invited Peter—a school friend who lives in the neighborhood—over to dinner. She served apple juice and natural corn chips as an appetizer. For our main course, we had chicken barbecued in a natural tamari and honey sauce, a big salad, and brown rice. For desert, we had fresh fruit. Peter really enjoyed himself—and saw that natural foods can be fun!

Share With Your Neighbors

Some of the pressure for your child to wander from the natural foods diet is bound to come from the neighbors themselves—from Jackie's mom or dad. Nevertheless, you can still enlist their support in keeping the junk food out of your child's diet. It all depends on how you approach them.

"Mrs. Smith, I really don't want Kristin eating all that junk you people eat. I'm convinced you're all going to die an early death from eating that stuff! I think you're wrong to eat that kind of food, so don't feed Kristin any of it when she's at your house."

Or ... you can try another approach.

"Mrs. Smith, I want to ask you for your help and support. We've been trying to stick to a natural foods diet because we've found we feel better when we eat natural foods. Kristin's schoolwork has improved, she has fewer colds, and I'm able to get a lot more work done. Kristin has been really receptive to the changes, and we're trying very hard, but I've never done anything like this before and I'm feeling my way through it. I think I can do it, but I know I'm going to need all the help I can get. I'd like to ask for your help in making sure Kristin eats only natural foods ... and, oh, by the way, here's this loaf of whole wheat bread I just baked this morning. It's Kristin's favorite recipe."

Don't Be a Salesperson for Natural Foods

If you try the first approach, naturally, you're going to get more doors slammed in your face than a vacuum cleaner salesman.

The second approach may work wonders—but even then, I must caution you against coming on too strong. Don't be a salesperson for your diet. You don't want the neighbors to have the following reaction when they see you coming.

"Oh, God, here she comes again with another loaf of her bread. It's good, but she never brings the bread without talking for 45 minutes about how wonderful natural foods are and how we should all be on natural foods. Oh, dear, she's headed this way, and I've got to get the cleaning and pick up the kids and make a salad for tonight's dinner! I think I'll just pretend I'm not home!"

Try to touch people on a human level—a level that goes deeper than beliefs and facts about the relative benefits of one kind of diet over another. Talk about and share with your neighbors some things that everyone can relate to—human things.

One of the best ways you can get someone to open up and really listen to you is to share with them some important, deep feelings and experiences you've had. Share your inner self, your fears and hopes. When you do this, they are more likely to let down their guard and really make an effort to understand what you're saying and support your goals as far as they can.

Tell a story about yourself. Tell them why you got into natural foods in the first place. Most people get into natural foods for really human reasons, from experiencing illness or healing. There's a big difference between sharing a story that begins with "I was sick ..." and one that begins with "The best diet in the world is ..." or ... "I'm not sick anymore and you shouldn't be either ... ."

Tell them what natural foods do *for you*—not what they can do for them. You don't have to share your deepest fears and experiences. You can start with something as simple as how you've found natural foods taste better. "Before, everything I ate tasted like cardboard. Now it tastes so good, I wonder why I'm not putting on weight."

The key word is *share*. You can share information about your experiences on a human level, and you can share the food itself. "Won't you come over for lunch ... or brunch ... or tea ... or dinner?"

If you share on a human level, and talk about things everyone can relate to, you will reach people. You may be surprised to find allies where you didn't expect to find them: "Gee ... that sounds like a great idea. You know, I've been waiting for just the right time to get *my* family on a natural foods diet, too. I'm so fed up with all this processed food! Now that I know you're doing this, I know I have someone to back me. Would you be interested in car-pooling to the nearest natural foods store?"

What If My Neighbor's House Is Junk Food City?

Naturally, you're not always going to get such a positive, supportive response. How do you handle the "worst case" situation, where your neighbor's house is Junk Food City? The first thing you do is sit down and have a talk with your child. Explain that Mrs. Smith simply does not feel the same way about food as you do. And then:

"I'm just going to have to ask you not to have any snacks over at their house. If you're hungry, you're big enough to come home and have a snack before you go over there. Always eat here first. And if you should get hungry after you're out playing with Jackie, then you're to come back here and have something to eat. That's the rule we're going to follow."

I believe that you do have the right and responsibility to set down certain rules and expect your child to follow them. (Of course, you also have a right to expect that the rules will be broken from time to time. We have a chapter coming up that will tell you just how big a hickory stick you should buy when your daughter comes home and tells you that Jackie's mom served up some chemically-processed sugar concoction that was just *irresistible!*)

But while we're on the subject of making rules and expecting that they will be honored—the same goes for your neighbors. While there's always the possibility that your neighbors will totally ignore your request for help and support, it's more likely they will get the message. Parents are generally attuned to each other's special rules. If Jackie's parents don't want Jackie riding her bike in the street, Joanie's mother will keep an eye on Jackie when the child is riding her bike in the neighborhood—even though Joanie, herself, *races* bicycles in her after-school hours.

Pressure on Teens Is the Greatest

Dealing with the peer pressure on a teenager is more difficult than dealing with it on younger children. With younger children, you can enlist the support of their friends' parents and even the teachers in their school, but teens pride themselves on their independence from these influences—even though the influences are still there.

Teens seem to be more affected by what's going on with their peers, too. They're very conscious of their social lives. They derive a great deal of their self-esteem from social activity, and their social lives are dependent on what their peers think of them. They, therefore, tend to be very conservative when it comes to acting independently of their peers.

Nevertheless, you can still turn peer pressure to your advantage, and in much the same way that you do it with younger children.

Focus your teenagers' attention on what the natural foods diet has done for her. If she can look at herself and see that her complexion is better, her hair has a healthier texture and body, and her schoolwork and athletic activities are more satisfying—then her self-esteem is being nourished. She will be better equipped to handle peer pressure.

You can still have your daughter's friends over for meals and snacks to demonstrate that natural foods can be even better tasting than junk food, and you can encourage your teen to share with her friends the *human* story behind your conversion to natural foods. Kids will generally understand, and support your teen in her efforts.

Teens really want to participate in what their friends are doing, so the junk food problem can come to a head when the gang wants to drive down to the local fast food restaurant and hang out. Fortunately, most fast food restaurants now offer salads, fruit juices, and other natural items on their menus. It's possible for your teen to hang out with the group and still stick to natural foods.

Naturally, there will be times when some of her friends won't totally support her. There are going to be times when they say, "Aww, c'mon, have a piece of cake! One slice won't hurt you! What's the matter with you?"

We all know that there are a lot worse things than birthday cake that teens can be tempted with these days, and I think it's important that we keep this problem in perspective. Even so, I do believe that the pressures on teens to "C'mon, have some of this. One won't hurt you!"

are basically the same, regardless of what "this" happens to be. The child's ability to say "I'm not going to do that!" and *know the reason why* derives from the same healthy self-esteem—whether the item in question is a piece of birthday cake, a can of beer, or a drug.

My daughter, Kristin, has helped me a lot in writing this book. I thought it would be a good idea to get her opinion directly on some of the problems we've tried to deal with in this chapter, so I've asked Kristin some questions and recorded her answers just as she gave them.

What was the biggest problem for you in changing your diet to natural foods?

"Going over to friends' houses and seeing them eat junk food and wanting some of it. I felt like I was the only person eating natural foods! It was hard to say no, and it's still hard to say no—especially when you see some other people eating something. I still like certain types of non-health foods. And I will eat them ... occasionally."

How do you deal with the response of your friends?

"They're basically understanding. A lot of people are starting to like natural foods more. They'll ask me what I'm eating and kind of look at it strangely, but most of the time they'd like to try it."

Do you ever find yourself in the position of having to justify your food preferences?

"Sometimes. I just say I tend to get sick easier if I eat junk food. It's true. If I eat too much unnatural food, I really don't feel that well. So I do find myself watching what I eat when I'm not home."

If you had to convince someone of the benefits of your diet, what would you say?

"I'd say that I feel pretty good when I'm on natural foods, but that when I eat other food, I don't feel that well. It's true. When I go away to camp every summer, I'm exposed to unnatural food—and I do tend to get more colds. Also, you can really taste the chemicals in junk food. When I eat natural foods, I don't get an awful taste in my mouth.

Do you see different families taking different approaches to change their diets to natural foods?

"Sure. Every family has a different viewpoint as they switch to natural foods. To some, sugar isn't that bad. Others eat lots of vegetables, but white rice is OK to them. Some take it slowly; some fast. I've noticed that people who have suffered heart attacks and other serious diseases tend to make drastic changes."

Any natural foods you don't like?

"Sure. Veggie burgers. Blah!"

Ever go for fast-food hamburgers?

"Sure. Once in a while."

What are your favorite natural foods?

"Fruits and vegetables. Brown rice. Fruit juices. Trail mixes. Lots of things! Pippin apples are my favorite!"

If you could say anything you want about natural foods, what would it be?

"I'd say give them a try. Not just for a week, either. You have to try it a little longer than that. See how you feel after a while. It's made a lot of changes in people that I know. Good changes."

Special Activities

Have a Party

Your child's birthday party is an excellent opportunity to show all her friends just how much fun natural foods can be. In fact, a party is such a good way to have fun with natural foods, why wait for your child's birthday to roll around? Have a natural foods tasting party *right away*! In either case, you can allow your child to help you select the menu.

Shopping

Take your child to a convenience market. Note the lack of natural foods and the "down mood" of the place. Then take her to a supermarket, natural foods store, and farm market. Ask her about the differences among the stores. Is there a relationship between the kind of food sold in the store and the feelings, attitudes, moods, and facial expressions of the people you see there?

Experiment

Young children really enjoy this one, and it's an excellent way to demonstrate that the properties of the food we eat do have a significant effect on our ... well ... on our "output." Go out to your garden and capture some snails. Put one snail in each of three jars. (Make sure the lids have holes in them!) Shred three pieces of construction paper— one red, one blue, one green or yellow, and put one color of paper in each jar, for each snail to eat. You will notice that the snails' droppings will be the same color as the construction paper they are raised on. From this experiment, you can demonstrate that what we eat does affect our body—all the way from one end to the other. Artificial colors (and flavors and preservatives) don't simply "disappear" when we eat them.

Gardening

Grow sunflowers. There is no more impressive plant that is so easy to grow. Just be sure you plant the seeds in a place that will allow for eight-foot flowers to grow! Your child will love showing off these beautiful giants to her friends, and the seeds are one of the most nutritious natural foods in existence!

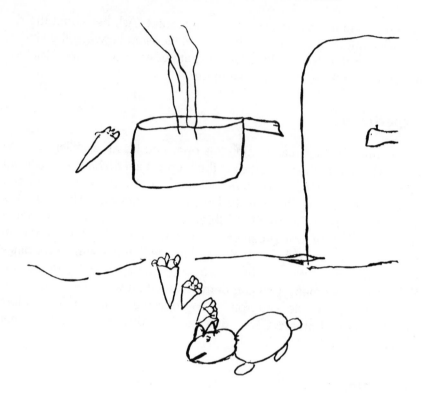

Carrots

Go to the store and buy 5 bunches of carrots. If you have a bunny, you give one to the bunny. Put the rest in the refrigerator, except one; and that you cook.

You cut it up in little round circles. Cut off the green stuff that the bunny likes to eat and chop that into little pieces. Now, both the green stuff and the orange circles are in the pan. Put it in the oven with one stick of butter, and cook it for 16 minutes.

Serve this with Kool Aid. Any leftovers you can give to the bunny.

Sandra Pagati

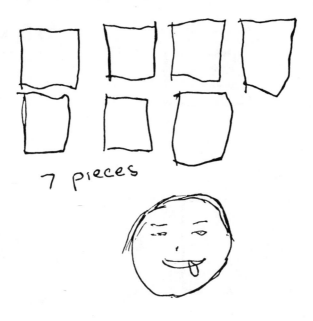

7 pieces

Seven French Toast

Put eggs and milk in a bowl. Mix it up. Put the bread in the mix. Put it in the oven for 1 minute. Take it out and put butter and syrup on it.

This recipe is called "Seven French Toast" 'cuz I can eat seven pieces.

Mark Burgos

But the kids on TV say

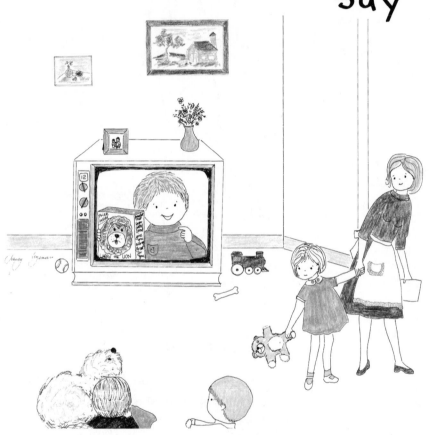

It's great and good for me!

10

You can read every book on nutrition and health and talk to your child about it until you're blue in the face ...

You can go out and get a Ph.D. in nutrition and teach your child everything you know ...

You can "start with yourself" and eliminate every ounce of junk from your house ...

You can enlist every neighbor within six miles in your natural foods revolution ...

You can make sure every in-law and relative knows that your child does not accept junk food ...

In short, you can win *every* battle there is to win ...

But there's no way you're going to keep your child from finding himself absolutely mesmerized before the dancing colors on a television screen selling junk food:

Greasy, salty fast food ...

Sugar-coated, candy breakfast cereals ...

Manufactured snack food ...

Soda pop ...

Chewing gum ...

Candy bars ...

And every ounce of it, the authoritative voice-over assures you, is "nutritious," "good for you," "part of a well-balanced diet," or "loaded with energy."

Of course, you know better. Even your *child* knows better, too.

But there's something irresistible about those commercials. TV ads really *motivate* people—especially little people. I can still remember Kristin singing the jingles one after the other as she got ready for school and went on her way every morning.

I can also remember her suddenly "waking up" in the middle of an otherwise uneventful shopping trip—and asking for the Choco-sweets or the Frosted Fancy Flakes the *very second* her eyes spotted the packages in the cereal aisle of the supermarket.

How many mothers absolutely *dread* turning the corner on the cereal aisle when their son or daughter is along because they know the child is going to make it very hard to get through the aisle without putting some of that heavily advertised junk in the cart?

And I know several parents—including myself—who have at times just taken the path of least resistance. When you're tired after a long day—or tired *in anticipation* of a long day!—you don't want to be bugged by this child making a scene in the middle of the market because you won't put the Choco-sweets in the cart.

If it will shut him up and let you get your shopping done ... *why not*? After all, you don't have to serve him the stuff. Once you get home with it, you can *hide it* somewhere.

Then the morning comes when you're in a hurry, and there's no time to prepare the toast and fruit your little boy loves, so ... *at least you can shove some Choco-sweets into him.*

And didn't the commercial assure you that Choco-sweets are—when eaten with milk—"part of a nutritious breakfast?"

Sure it did. So you can fly out the door heaving an astronomical sigh of relief because, Thank God, your child has had an "adequate breakfast!"

This little scenario takes place millions of times every day. TV commercials work their devilish magic on all of us, one way or the other—either by influencing our children or planting little convenient "facts" here and there in our minds. It doesn't have to be that way. We don't have to allow the commercials to tell our children (and us!) what foods to like, want, buy, and eat, and we don't have to chuck the tube out the window to do it, either. We can prepare our children to deal effectively with the influence of television commercials in much the same way that we prepare them to deal with peer pressure.

When I look at a TV commerical for junk food, toys, clothes, or anything else a child is likely to want or need, I see an incredible amount of peer pressure being put on the child viewer. I see one group after another of absolutely wonderful-looking children having *such a great time* eating this or that cereal, playing with this or that toy, or going to this or that amusement park.

And don't those children in the commercial look like a really great gang to hang out with! They're having *so much fun!* It's going to be awfully hard for a child to resist wanting to be accepted by them, to be just like they are and have the things they have—in particular, whatever it happens to be that they're selling.

Those children—and their animated friends—on the screen literally *scream out* to our children: "Hey, c'mon and join the fun! Join *us! Jump on our bandwagon!* Everybody's doing it! Why don't you?"

Our children are no less status-conscious than we are, but where our desire for status is satisfied by a fancy car, designer clothes, and other such stylish items we see advertised, their desires are satisfied by the products they see their "TV friends" enjoying. The fact that they can actually *have* what they see in the magic world inside the television has tremendous appeal to them.

The people who create those commercials plan it that way.

I know ... because when Kristin was between the ages of three and six years old she appeared in several commercials—for pizza, dolls, and cosmetics. For some of those thirty-second commercials, she would have to be in the studio for more than four days, until it was just the way the director wanted it. I can still hear the director telling her over and over again: "Smile, Kristin! Look happy!"

In preparing this chapter, I spoke with two professional advertising executives (Doug Stone and Richard Holmes)—men who have been in the advertising business for years, and who have been educated and trained to create effective ads and commercials.

It was a real eye-opener for me, even though I've been "in the business" myself for several years, both through my natural food markets and Kristin's involvement in TV commercials. I asked them to tell me how these commercials are conceived and what the creators have in mind, aside from selling as many boxes of Choco-sweets as possible.

The "trick" or aim of a TV commercial is to get the viewer to "get the message," or duplicate the thought of the ad. Even though the commercial may seem to be a regular three-ring circus of activity, there are always four or five very specific messages the ad wants the viewer to take away with him.

The advertisers are very good at meeting the audience on its psychological-developmental level. The admen call this "meeting the kids' sense of reality." They do this by portraying a world that the child can really "get into," a world the child will *want* to live in. They fill the screen with scenes, people, activities, and *themes* that appeal to children.

The scenes are happy scenes, intriguing scenes, fascinating scenes, or colorful scenes. The characters (more about those lovable demons later!) are cute, attractive, friendly, happy, and—above all—trustworthy. The activities are all great fun, and the themes are too good to be true—and too devilishly clever to ignore. They include: *All life is a game. Nobody ever loses. Everybody always wins.*

Can you blame a child for wanting a piece of *that* action? Can you blame him for being attracted to the *single item* most visibly and demonstrably associated with that action in the ad—*the product?*

The other themes that advertising executives spoke of as "primary motivators" were adventure and fantasy. "Let's go on an adventure, kids!" "Let's enjoy this fantasy!" "*Let's go on this mission that will be filled with adventure, fantasy, and fun!*"

Of course, the child cannot jump into the tube and go on the adventure with the characters, but he can do the next best thing. He can buy the product they take along with them and *imagine* he's along for the ride.

It can get pretty scary when you start to understand how the advertisers have the art of persuasion and selling down to a science—an exact science that expertly manipulates our children's desires for fun, adventure, and acceptance.

But save your scaries, because what your child sees on the TV screen accounts for only half of the advertiser's marketing skill. The other half goes into the design of the product package. You can't deal effectively with the influence of TV ads unless you understand the psychology behind the *packaging* of the junk food advertised on TV.

The basic "buy this" message of the TV commercial is reinforced and finally "brought home" by two major elements of the package that also appear in the commercial—what the admen call the "cons" and the "credible entities." The credible entities are the characters and people who appear on the packages, and the cons are the messages they deliver.

And you thought the cereal manufacturers just casually decided to hire some poor starving artist to "come up with a pretty box" for their product? No way. They know that no amount of skill could ever give your child a sensation of what's actually *in* the box. They can tell him it's sweet and delicious and so-o-o good for him, but they can't sell it to him by giving him an actual taste. Since they can't sell him on what's *in* the box, they have to sell him ... the box.

Years of research and experience have taught them that the package, more often than not, makes the difference between whether or not the product sells. They spend *millions* of dollars on the best advertising design and market research skills that money can buy to come up with just the right cast of characters to deliver just the right script of cons to get you and your child to feel good about buying that *box* of Choco-sweets. The Choco-sweets themselves are inconsequential. All that junk tastes pretty much the same. They know that. It's just something to fill the box. Your child is attracted to—and you're buying—that biggest, brightest-colored, deepest-hued, totally Madison-Avenued box!

(The box *is* actually worth more than the junk food inside. Not only does more care and skill go into it, but it's nutritionally better, too, at least for *rats*. An enterprising researcher found that rats fared better when they were fed the boxes than when they ate the cereal inside!)

Cast of Characters

Take a stroll down the cereal aisle of the supermarket. Direct your attention to the lower shelves—the ones that are on eye-level for a child. All those brightly-colored boxes of junk cereal aren't placed on that shelf by accident. The supermarket staff receives explicit instructions to put those boxes right where your child's eyes will fall upon Larry the Lion and Admiral Sugar Corn and Rainbow Randy the Fruit Bunny and Doughnut Dog and the Frosty Fairy and *all* those syrupy sweet characters you see every Saturday morning selling junk food cereal.

Look for a box of "kid cereal" *without* a cheerful character.

You won't find one.

Fruit Bunny and Larry the Lion and all their friends are the "credible entities" created by the admen to sell the products to your children. Young children (and many adults, too!) relate to these characters. They believe them. They're entertained by them, so that makes them OK, trustworthy, and *credible*.

Dull, drab boxes don't move the merchandise. Colorful, adventurous, fun characters do. So here's Fruit Bunny. His whiskers are dragging and he's hopping up and down asking your child to *please* try this cereal, because it's "good and good for you." Because "it's fun!"

Consider for a moment the awesome *power* animated characters can have. If you have trouble doing that, consider what Mickey Mouse did for Walt Disney. Got the picture?

The cereal manufacturers couldn't buy Mickey Mouse to sell their products, but they realized they could *create their own* characters to their own specifications. If you watch enough Saturday morning TV with your child, you'll be treated to one exciting, fantastic, comical, fun adventure after another—interrupted only by the actual programs.

Watch these characters. They're real heroes. They're adventurous, brave, vulnerable, comical, a bit mischievous, never-complacent, and cute. They're good guys through and through, and they're *always having lots of fun*.

Children really eat that stuff up—whether they ever taste the cereal or not. But the pressure to please go out and buy the cereal is there, created by this lovable little Fruit Bunny or this great big—but so very friendly—Larry the Lion. When your child sees the very same character greeting him at eye level in the syrupmarket (Oops! I mean supermarket ...)—*the very same wonderful character he saw on TV!*—the character literally comes to life once again. The attraction is incredibly strong.

Is that so hard to understand? You know how thrilled we are when we get a chance to be on TV. And aren't we all just simply enthralled when we have the opportunity to meet someone who is a "TV star"? How thrilling it would be to actually have a TV star come home with us and spend some time and eat breakfast with us! If such a star offered to come home with us and do that, would we quibble if he wanted us to serve his favorite cereal?

Of course not!

Keep in mind that our younger children—the ones most susceptible to this kind of advertising—have not established very clear boundaries in their minds between fantasy and reality. Rainbow Randy the Fruit

Bunny and the Frosty Fairy are *very real* to them—even more real than the stars of your favorite TV show are to you.

Larry the Lion and Doughnut Dog are on the screen and the box to do a lot more than appear cute and lovable and have adventures. Their job is to sell cereal, and they do that by delivering several skillfully created "cons" during the course of the commercial—or while your eyes skim over the cereal box itself.

They tell you how the Choco-sweets are part of a balanced breakfast. They don't tell you that they are the devitalized, worthless part of a balanced breakfast, the part that weighs the other parts down.

They tell you that the cereal is fortified with lots of vitamins. They don't tell you that you'll need more vitamins than you can get in the whole box to make up for the nutritional damage done by eating a single bowl of sugar-coated junk. They don't dare tell you about all the things that have been removed from the original grain.

The cons tell you that the cereal has been "approved by our panel of experts." Cons like this usually appear on the cereal box next to a quacky-looking doctor-type, or a child dressed up to look like he's playing doctor, or a bunch of smiling children wearing offical-looking spectacles.

Even the official-looking list of ingredients contains a masterful con. Aware that label readers look first to see how far towards the front of the list "sugar" appears, cereal manufacturers have learned to *fractionate* the sugars. What you see is sugar appearing as number two or three or four on the list, but later on down the list you'll find dextrose, corn sugar, fructose, brown sugar, turbinado sugar, sucrose, levulose, maltose, or any of a half-dozen other types of sugar.

One of the most popular cons is the "free surprise inside." How many dozens of boxes of junk cereal did we all make our parents buy just so we could have the exquisite adventure of searching for that treasure inside the box, hidden amidst all that crunchy sweet stuff we really couldn't care less about?

Then there are the endless contests ... games ... sweepstakes ... educational come-ons ... .

If you examine a con, you'll always come to either a dead end in logic (This is the best cereal that ever was!) or an outright lie (Choco-sweets are good for you!). A con is just what the word itself means in our society—a promise that isn't meant to be fulfilled. In other words, a lie.

By the way, it wasn't my idea to use the word "con" for those little statements on cereal boxes. Con is the word used by the admen themselves!

Beat the Admen at Their Own Game!

The techniques the admen use to con children into wanting their products are serious business, but the best way to beat the admen is to *make a game out of it.* You want to expose the commercial and the package for what they are—come-ons. You want to analyze and discuss the advertising messages, the claims, the quality of the product, the characters, and how the product fits in—or doesn't fit in—with your natural foods diet. If you want your child to get *your* message, you've got to make the process *more fun than the commercials themselves.*

So make a game out of it. Remember, one of the irresistible themes of the commercials is "Life is fun and everyone's a winner." Structure the game so that your child is always the winner. Try making a game out of exploring your child's attraction to the commercial. Ask him why the commercial is interesting. Why do you enjoy this commercial? What are the characters doing? What does the cereal (or other product) have to do with what the characters are doing? Why did the people who made this commercial put Larry the Lion (or whomever) in there? What does Larry say about the cereal? Does Larry tell you about all the sugar that's in the cereal? Why doesn't Larry tell you about how all the sugar and chemicals can be harmful?

You can examine all the characters and cons with your child until he figures out the whole game. See how many cons he can uncover all by himself. Then, congratulate him for understanding what is really going on in the TV commercials. That makes him the winner, because he can still enjoy the shenanigans of the characters. Only now, he'll know that *extra secret mischief* they're up to, and *he* won't be fooled!

The younger child will be less able to distinguish between the fantasy cartoon world of the character and the real, flesh-and-blood world, but with an older child, say one who is eight or older, you can begin to explore what is actually going on in the commercials in a more analytical manner. Not only can you explore with him his own responses to the characters and their cons, but you can go behind the scenes of the fantasy world. You can talk about how the children in the commercials are really actors who are paid to appear happy and smile as they eat their Frosty Freaky Flakes.

To take the game a step further, you cannot only go behind the scenes of the commercial, but also look into the manufacturing process by which a perfectly good grain is turned into the sugary junk advertised in the commercial.

You and your child have "won the game" when the TV commercials and supermarket come-ons no longer make him want to "join the fun" by eating the product—when he understands and really feels that the cartoons and the characters are there to entertain him, not instruct him in how to feed and take care of his body.

Still, There Comes a Time ...

Admen will be admen ... and children will be children. Goodness knows, both the admen and the children are extremely good at what they do. There may come a time—even after you've had a lot of fun exposing Fruit Bunny for the con-artist that he is—when the child just wants to "try some."

But parents will also be parents, and we have a right to be good at what *we* do, too. There comes a time when it's not only your right, but your responsibility, to be firm. Don't be afraid to say no. There's nothing wrong in saying: "We're not going to have Choco-sweets (anymore)."

I know one family who solved this problem of TV commercials right from the start. It was a hard and fast rule in their house that they would *never buy any food advertised on TV.*

That may be going a little bit too far. After all, the day is rapidly approaching when we'll see Grover the Whole Grain Groundhog telling us all about how good truly natural cereals can be.

Special Activities

Make Your Own Commercials. Once you've analyzed the commercials for junk food, the best way to continue the game is to use that new knowledge to expose the "secrets" of the junk food hucksters. You and your child can do this by making a satirical commercial for the junk food.

Help your child write a "script" for a commercial in which Larry the Lion or the Frosty Fairy or the Fruit Bunny *tells the truth* about Choco-sweets, or whatever his favorite cereal happens to be. Make sure you warn the unsuspecting viewers of the health dangers of junk food. Expose all the false claims the real commercials have made.

Then, you and your child can act out the script. Or, you can lie in wait for Fruit Bunny and Captain Corn on Saturday morning ... and when they appear on the TV screen, you can turn the sound down and supply *your own* satirical lines while they cavort happily unsuspecting on the screen.

This game is fun, and it serves a very useful purpose. By taking over the voice of the characters and telling the truth about their products, your child will substitute *the truth* in his mind whenever the characters come on the screen. He will never "hear" their message without *his own* also coming through louder and clearer. Larry the Lion and Fruit Bunny and the rest will never be the same again for him—thank goodness!

You can also make commercials for your own wholesome cereals. After you've exposed the secrets of junk food with your satirical commercials, you can go on to "selling" your own natural cereals—granola, whole grains, etc. Start by making a list of all the good things you can say about the food: its nutritional value, taste, convenience, and so forth.

Next, you'll need a spokesperson. That's right. You now get to *create your own character* to sell your "product." Remember, your "credible entity" should be trustworthy, adventurous, mischievous, cute, brave, and vulnerable. You and your child can have lots of fun coming up with adventures for your characters.

And don't forget the "cons." After all, if the junk food manufacturers can get away with saying things like "approved by a panel of experts," why can't you?

Making your own commercials gives you and your child lots of opportunities for artwork. He may not be able to actually animate a cartoon or videotape a live-action commercial, but he can draw a series of scenes and actions that can be strung together to make what is called a "story board." Professional cartoonists always make a story board before getting down to work on the actual cartoon animation.

Your child can also decorate a cereal box of his own. Using the same principles as the admen, you can create a "package" for your natural food with lots of colors and happy characters having lots of fun. You can add the "cons," too.

Cooking. Since breakfast cereals seem to be the area where junk food TV commercials concentrate, I suggest your cooking activities for this chapter center on the granola recipe and some of the nutritious bread recipes you'll find in Appendix B.

Remember the Fun. Lots of TV commercials sell children on how much fun it is to go out and have a Greaseburger and Fatty Fries at the local fast food restaurant. These commercials use the same strategies as commercials for breakfast cereals.

Remember, it's not so much the fast food hamburgers or chicken drumsticks on which the children are sold. What turns on children is the experience of going somewhere that is accepted with people they love. You can duplicate this experience without going to a fast food restaurant by going to a natural foods restaurant or going on a picnic. Several fast food restaurants have responded to the growing desire for natural foods, so you may find salads and other wholesome entrees you and your children can enjoy.

If you remember that the lure of TV commercials consists of fun, adventure, and acceptance—and you make up your mind that you are going to supply these necessities to your child, instead of the television characters and their products—you and your family should have no problem warding off the influence of Larry the Lion, Fruit Bunny, Captain Corn, Frosty Fairy, and the rest of the menagerie when they come calling.

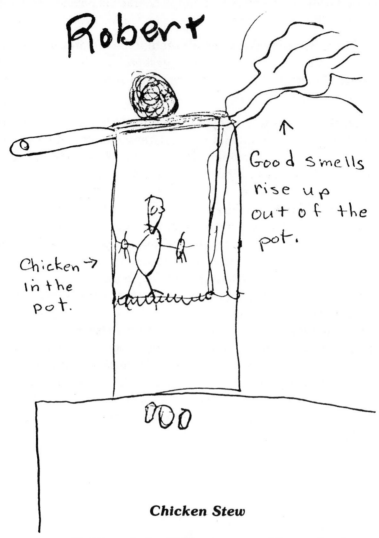

Chicken Stew

Put the whole chicken in a pot. (It's not dead yet.) Put in 2 cups of water, 6 carrots and 4 pieces of celery. Put in a shake of salt and 4 cups of pepper. Cook all this for 2 whole hours. Serve it in a dish.

I don't cut the chicken, I just eat it the way it's built.

Robert Abdulla

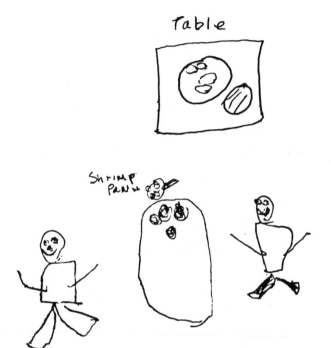

Fried Shrimp

Put 4 shrimp in a pan that has a little bit of burning up oil in it. Cook them for I don't know how long and then turn them over and do the same thing on the other side.

Serve this with asparagus. But the dish has to be separated.

Kevin Masuda

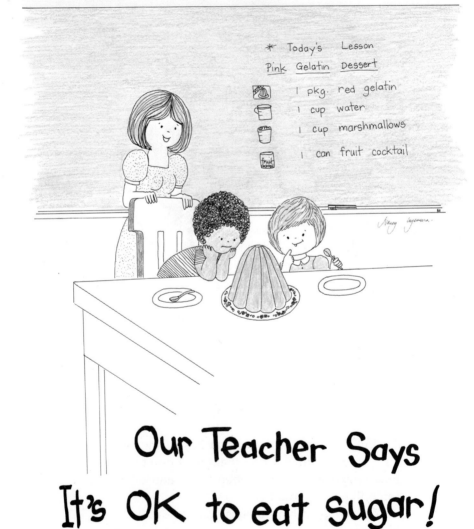

Our Teacher Says
It's OK to eat sugar!

11

We've all experienced the times when our child comes home and says:

"Mommie, we made pink gelatin dessert in school today!"

"Mommie, teacher showed us how to make sugar pudding today. Can I make some for you tonight?"

"Mommie, they put a new vending machine in the cafeteria today. I can put my own quarters in and get a candy bar!"

"Mommie, the cafeteria started serving a new dessert today— Sugar Rockets!"

"Mommie, *teacher says it's OK to eat white sugar!*"

I've been on both sides of these dilemmas. For seventeen years I was a schoolteacher. To this day, I feel so guilty about my early days as a teacher, when I taught my little, unsuspecting schoolchildren to make sugary, artificial, chemical-laden gelatin dessert ... when I showed them how to make sugar pudding ... when we used white flour by the ten-pound bag on some days!

I didn't know any better. My goal was to teach them about measurements, eating and cooking habits, and working in teams. When the lesson did have something to do with nutrition, I taught them the very same misinformation I had learned in college. The four food groups were all you needed to know about nutrition as far as I was concerned.

121

Of course, my awareness changed after I was sick. After I learned the value of natural foods, I did share my new knowledge with my classes. We ground our own grain and learned about whole wheat and honey and the hazards of junk food. We even learned how to grow our own sprouts.

Our children's exposure to junk food at school is one of the toughest problems to tackle. There are really *three* problems wrapped up in the one package called "school." One, your child is exposed to peer pressure from the other children. Two, your child is exposed to the influence of the teacher, who may or may not know beans about the difference between a sprout and a doughnut. Three, your child is exposed to the junk food itself—in the cafeteria and in the vending machines.

Kristin is almost ready to go off to college, and, believe me, she's had her share of junk food junkies for teachers. Her school cafeterias have hardly been models of natural foods kitchens either, so I've done my share of facing this problem. As with other problems having to do with resistance from other people, the best route to success is through honest communciation and sharing. Level with your child's teacher(s). Enlist their help. Offer to share your experience and knowledge with the class.

Leveling with your child's teacher may not be the easiest thing to do. We relinquish so much of our parental authority and responsibility to the school system these days, that we're often uncomfortable when we try to reclaim some of it. Sometimes there is an institutional barrier that prevents people from communicating, sharing, and helping one another. More often, it's the *fear and anticipation* of the barrier that slows us down.

You don't have to approach the teacher with a defensive attitude. Remember what we said earlier about affirming the positive. Put your attention on the positive, not the negative possibilities. If you go into a meeting with the teacher anticipating resistance, chances are you'll find it.

It's also not such a good idea to go to the teacher with your sword drawn and your cannons loaded for action. Your child's teacher is going to be even more sensitive than your neighbors if you come on too forcefully. If you come out swinging, the teacher's first reaction is going to be to defend herself. Then, if you ever want to get your point across, you'll have to first undo all the resistance caused by that first, hasty attack.

Think about what your goal is. You really don't want to *convert* the teacher, do you? Let me assure you that it's not necessary to do so. It's enough that the teacher *acknowledges* your goals and habits regarding food and promises to support you and your child in reaching those goals.

When I say level with the teacher, I mean you can go in with the attitude that the teacher is going to be understanding of different ways of life. Lots of parents have no problem at all going to a teacher and saying, "Joanie has to have an operation next month, so we'd like to make some special arrangements to have her work sent home for a couple of weeks while she's convalescing ... ."

It's even easier to go to a teacher and say, "We are making an effort to change our family diet. We want to get rid of as much junk as we can and, you know, I feel Joanie's schoolwork might improve as much as her health has if we can keep her on the best possible natural foods diet. *I'd like to be able to count on your help and support in this effort. Joanie herself has tried really hard, too."*

Chances are excellent—in fact, I'm willing to *bet*—that the teacher's reply will be something along the lines of, "Just let me know what I can do to help out." That is the open door you are looking for. It's your opportunity to share with the teacher your specific desires and goals for your child's diet. You can say something like: "Thank you. We really do need your help because we eat a different way at home. We don't use any white sugar, or any white flour, or any foods with artificial additives ... etc."

You should be clear about—and ready to communicate—exactly what you expect from the teacher in the way of support and help. I feel that just receiving the teacher's acknowledgement and agreement is the most important step. From that point on, the teacher is aware of your child's specialness. When the class is involved in some kind of food situation, the teacher will be "on notice" that your child's habits are different from those of the rest of the class. And if the other students—or the situation itself—puts pressure on your child, the teacher's support can make all the difference.

Of course, the teacher's responses to your plea might be, "I'd like to help ... but I don't really believe in natural foods myself." This is not necessarily a closed door. It may mean only that you cannot expect the teacher to hold back on the sugar pudding lessons and Sugar Rockets for snacks, but you still have a right to ask for support. And you, of course, still have the responsibility to make sure the teacher is aware of your standards for your child.

I'm reminded of the story of a very feisty young mother I knew some years ago. She was quite particular about what she allowed her children to eat. She went to the principal of the school and said, "My children can eat only such and such ... and I would like your permission to talk to the people in the cafeteria about this."

She got permission, and her next stop was the cafeteria. She talked to every person who worked in that cafeteria and made sure they all knew who her children were and what they were allowed—and not allowed—to eat. They were to get the hot entree and salad, but no desserts, chocolate milk, or white bread.

It took her months of going back and repeating her requests to the cafeteria staff, since they did not all get the message the first time ... or the second ... or even the third time she explained it. And, of course, school cafeterias are very busy places. The personnel have to work very fast to keep the lines moving.

But they eventually got the message. They knew she meant business—and they respected her for it. And ... *other mothers joined with her to improve the cafeteria food.*

Teachers Need (And Love!) All the Help They Can Get

One magical day you're going to sit down with your child's teacher to "level with her" regarding your dietary rules and regulations and ... lo and behold! She'll reply with something like this: "Why, I'm into natural foods, too. I'm so glad you came in to talk about this. I've been thinking about teaching the children about nutrition and health and natural foods ... ."

This is your golden opportunity to offer *your* help. As a matter of fact, you don't even have to wait to find a teacher who is "into" natural foods. You can offer your time and energy to help the teacher plan and execute lessons on food and nutrition: "I've been reading and studying nutrition quite a lot ... and I'd be happy to share some of my experiences with the class."

Even teachers who are not totally into natural foods may be very grateful for your help in giving a lesson on the health benefits of not eating white sugar and white flour. You could cap off a lesson like this with a tasting party of a whole wheat cake made with honey and other natural ingredients.

Children are really receptive to these little "vignette lessons." I've learned from the class tours I conduct through my markets—as well as from my seventeen years experience as a teacher—that children's eyes and ears are wide-open when they are on a special field trip outside the classroom. They are equally open to new information when a visitor comes into the classroom to share something with them.

My class tours of the markets are only about half-an-hour long, but those children are always left with several impressions and new bits of information about nutrition. I always hear about these impressions from *parents* and *teachers* in the days and weeks after the tours.

In one school in the ghetto of East Los Angeles, a complete nutrition education program grew out of the children's response to the class tour of one of my markets. Their appetites for learning were whetted, and they subsequently kept on asking questions about diet and health. Finally, their schoolteachers started a comprehensive program in the school to meet the demand.

A similar thing may very well happen after you give your capsule lesson on the dangers of white sugar or the joys of whole wheat flour. The children will want to know more. They'll ask the teacher questions. You may be asked back for another "demonstration" (read: "cake"). Before you know it, you will have converted the entire class—including the teacher!

I really believe that you'll find—as I have found—that many teachers are trying their best to improve the quality of the food in their schools. I've recently become acquainted with Susan Baumeister, a perceptual-motor specialist and physical education teacher for the Beverly Hills School District. Apparently, the affluence of a school district doesn't guarantee the best food for its students. The *Beverly Hills* school district regularly serves its students run-of-the-mill, garden variety, plain old junk food, including: canned fruits and vegetables, orange drink loaded with artificial chemicals and sugar, crunchy (greasy) cheese chips, artificial orange sherbet, and sugary gelatin dessert!

Sue has worked very hard to change all that and improve the cafeteria food. She's been motivated not only by her own experience and awareness about diet and health, but also by her observations that her students often displayed behavioral, perceptual, and coordination difficulties *after lunch!* Sue has proposed to the school board a number of activities designed not only to improve the food served in the Beverly Hills Schools but also to improve the nutritional education the students receive. She has also contacted several natural foods distributors and gone over her district's food requirements to find out just how much natural food they will need to order and how much it will cost.

Sue's proposals include:

1. Substituting natural foods for processed foods in the school lunch program.

2. Encouraging and providing information and/or classes in natural food planning and preparation for food service employees.

3. Planning a district-wide Health Day, which would include speakers, tasting booths, exhibits on alternatives to junk food, skits, art projects (collage of junk food wrappers, collage of natural foods, student-designed cookbooks) and a natural foods cooking contest. (See "Special Activities" at the end of this chapter for instructions on planning your own natural bake-off.)

4. Cooking natural foods in each classroom.

5. Starting a program of nutrition education for the entire school district, so every student would have the opportunity to learn about natural foods.

6. Organizing field trips to natural foods stores, farms, natural foods distributors, etc.

7. Publishing a newsletter bringing nutritional news and facts to students, parents, and teachers.

8. Forming parent-student committees to discuss diet and nutritional practices in the schools.

Sue's proposals are now being reviewed by the Beverly Hills school board. Sue is optimistic that her program will be adopted. She has the support of several families in the district. Many people—teachers, parents, students, and administrators—have demonstrated their support. (As this book goes to press, the Beverly Hills school board has not only agreed to review Sue's proposals, but has also allocated funds to analyze the nutritional content of cafeteria food and recommend improvements.)

Let Your Child Share and Tell

The other children are going to ask your child questions, too. Questions ranging from: "What's so bad about sugar? My mom let's me eat all the candy I want when I'm good!"—to—"Gee, that cake was sure good! Can I come over to your house and get some more?"

Chances are that the *teacher* may also begin to refer to your child for information about nutrition in a positive, cheerful manner. "Maybe Kristin can tell us something about sprouts?" Or, "Maybe Kristin can tell us why whole wheat is better than refined flour?"

You can prepare your child for these encounters the same way you prepare her to handle peer pressure from her friends. (See Chapter 9.) As in any educational endeavor, *attitude* is all-important. If you and your child approach people with the attitude that "Everyone who doesn't eat the same way we eat is going to get sick," then you'll be met with skepticism, defensiveness, and even hostility. But, if you and your child approach people with "This is what we've found works for us, and we'd like to share as much of our experience with you as we can," you'll be met with acceptance, receptiveness, and curiosity.

As far as I know, they still have "share and tell" in school. This gives your child a golden opportunity to share her experiences with natural foods—and to share some natural goodies, too, such as natural breakfast cereals, natural snacks, and natural desserts.

Children can bring in all kinds of things to "share and tell." Your child and some of her classmates can put together a satirical junk food commercial (see the previous chapter) and perform it for the class. Children love to put on little shows for their friends.

The Sara Sloan Story: You May Have To Overhaul the Entire School!

Let us not forget that schools are institutions, that institutions may become bureaucracies, and that bureaucracies seldom have the slightest regard for common sense. It's quite possible that you will run into the kind of situation a friend of mine did.

Sally's youngest daughter was in kindergarten. The children were required to bring in their own lunches when the school's kitchen closed down. The only rule was that they were not allowed to bring in any "candy." Sounds good so far—until you learn that "candy" did not exclude soda pop and sugar-filled cakes made with artificial colors and flavors and lots of air. Sally had excluded that kind of junk from her family's diet long ago—and her children had no problem with the change, so Sally packed fruit rolls made with a little bit of honey in her daughter's lunch. Her daughter came home with a note from the teacher repeating the school's rule that children not bring "candy" in their lunches.

Sally was flabbergasted. She called the teacher, who told her over the phone not to send candy in the child's lunch. Undaunted, Sally went straight to the school board. She explained to them that she was very concerned about what her children ate and that, in her opinion, a fruit roll made with all natural ingredients was certainly no more "candy" than the fake cakes and pies the other kids were allowed to bring to school. The school board relented and agreed that Sally's daughter could bring in the fruit rolls for lunch.

Sally was lucky in that she did not run into a stone wall of bureaucratic inertia. She was forceful and determined enough to bring her case "all the way to the supreme court" of her school district.

I hope we don't all need to go quite that far to make sure our children are protected from junk food while they're in school. Nevertheless, my advice is to go "right to the top" of your school district's administration if the teacher is not supportive.

If you and your child do run into a totally unreceptive and unsupportive attitude on the part of teachers and administrators—and I sincerely doubt that you will—you are left with two "worst case" alternatives. I shouldn't identify these two courses of action as alternatives, because that implies you should choose one and ignore the other. Actually, you should take the first course of action regardless of whether or not you take the second, and that course is the same as I recommended in my chapter on peer pressure from the neighborhood.

Treat a "junk food-saturated" school the same way you would a neighbor's house that was an incorrigible "junk food city." Make sure your child is well-fed before she goes off to school in the morning, pack her a nutritious lunch, and make sure she knows she has a marvelous natural foods snack waiting for her when she comes home.

The second alternative is to charge the bureaucracy head-on and try to work within the system to change it. Entire volumes have been written on this single subject, and my purpose in this book is to help you overcome human resistance on a person-to-person level, rather than on an institutional level.

I want to inspire you by assuring you that it *can be done*, and support you by pointing you in the direction of Sara Sloan, a woman who not only changed the food system in an entire school district—but who has made a career out of helping other people do the same in their school districts.

More than twenty years ago, Sara Sloan was head of the home economics department in a high school in Fulton County, Georgia. Sara became interested in the effects of food on health and learning ability. The more she read, the more convinced she became that a natural foods diet could improve behavior and learning ability among schoolchildren. Sara set about changing the food that was fed to schoolchildren in the Fulton County Schools, and today, Fulton County schoolchildren enjoy farm fresh natural produce, whole grain cereals, additive-free meats, and sugar-free desserts.

Results? The school system's standardized achievement test scores rose by at least an entire grade level after the change.

And Sara, who is now Director of Food and Nutrition Programs for the Fulton County Schools (Atlanta), proudly boasts: "We do not allow pornographic literature in our libraries and we will not allow pornographic foods in our kitchens."

Sara makes available to parents, school districts—anyone who is interested—several publications that are designed to help people get better food into their children and into their schools, including an invaluable newsletter called "Nutritional Parenting." I will mention some of her books in Appendix C, but here is her address, from which you can request more information, including her newsletter for parents: Sara Sloan, NUTRA, Box 13825, Atlanta, Georgia 30324.

I have recently had the privilege of serving on the Los Angeles County Board of Supervisors' Task Force on Nutrition and Behavior. Among other things, we have investigated the possibilities of improving the diets of children in the county's juvenile detention centers.

In connection with our work with the Task Force, Sue Epstein and I conducted a seminar on cooking natural foods. Most of the audience consisted of cooks from the various institutions run by the county— juvenile detention centers, jails, etc. Most of these cooks had never had any kind of nutritional education whatsoever. Many of them had once been cooks in the armed forces.

I was worried that we might be greeted with reticence and a wall of resistance, to put it mildly.

Instead, Sue and I were met with receptiveness and curiosity. They absolutely fell in love with natural food! They *all* said, "You know, the kids would really love this. But we don't know how to do it! Please give us more information, more seminars, more instruction, and more opportunities to make this kind of food for the kids!"

A couple of weeks later, we took some natural food down to the Kirby Juvenile Detention Home. We made totally natural sandwiches with whole wheat bread and sprouts. I made carob pudding. We had meatless chili, whole wheat buns, raw milk cheddar cheese, and natural oatmeal cookies.

Then we interviewed the children. In front of television cameras for a local station. Live.

The children all said, in one way or another: "We love it! Give us more of this wonderful food!"

Whenever someone tells me "It can't be done," I point them in the direction of Sara Sloan. And when they say, "Yeah, but the kids won't eat that stuff," or, "The cooks will never go for it," I tell them about the excitement and receptivity and enthusiasm we found at Kirby—and at the many other schools across the country that have successfully switched to natural foods.

All of these natural foods revolutions began with one dedicated, tenacious person who wanted the best food for his or her children.

Special Activities

Your daughter's school birthday party can be a "natural." Have her help you select, shop for, and prepare the natural goodies for the party. If your school has restrictions about bringing homemade food into the classroom, there is an abundance of packaged natural goodies available: fruit juice, cakes, cookies, ice cream, fresh fruit desserts, yogurt, natural snacks, trail mix, and granola, to name a few.

Lunches can be abundant with fun! One of the best ways for your child to deal with the curiosity of her friends about the "strange food" she brings for lunch is to encourage her to share some of it with her friends. When I knew a food was something extra-delicious that would attract attention, I always packed extra amounts for Kristin to share with her friends. I packed extra carrot cake, honey cake, carrot chips (when they first came out and were a real curiosity) and ... sprouts.

That's right, sprouts. One day Kristin went to school and had alfalfa sprouts hanging out of her sandwich. One child looked at this sandwich and the sprouts and was simply incredulous! "Kristin, are you eating grass?" she asked.

"No, alfalfa," Kristin replied.

The next day I packed an extra packet of alfalfa for Kristin's friend.

You and your child can have more fun with lunch if you approach it as a team effort. Allow your child to choose her menu for the week. She can then help you shop for and prepare the lunches.

Finally, I want to tell you about something I have always done for Kristin's lunch. Every day, I write Kristin a little note on a napkin or a piece of paper and slip it in her lunch. She tells me I'm the only mother who does that, and the other children really notice. There's a special meaning inside that lunch for her, even if she's not totally aware of it. It's not an ordinary lunch bag, by any means. The other children say, "Wow, you have a mother who does *that?*"

I keep the notes simple: "I'm proud of the way you handled the company yesterday."

"Love is having a daughter who always has a smile on her face!"

"I'm sorry you woke up unhappy this morning and we didn't have a chance to talk about it. We'll talk later, OK?"

"Don't forget, I'm picking you up early!"

I've even written notes to Kristin's friends.

"Dear Jane, Kristin told me you really enjoyed the cream cheese and olive sandwich yesterday. I'm so glad you did. Here are some carrot chips for you to try."

It takes hardly any time at all. At the most—on days when I've felt like writing Kristin a poem—five minutes. Sometimes, I will just scrawl a happy face picture on her napkin. I usually write it on her napkin, because I know that's something she will pick up and use, but there have been times when I've hidden it in the sandwich somewhere.

Today, I know Kristin is trying to take off a few pounds, so I wrote, "Good luck with your diet!"

(See Appendix B for more ideas on natural lunches and making lunches abundant with fun!)

Cooking Share and Tell. Do some research and plan meals of natural foods from countries your child is studying in school. She can later share the experience—and perhaps even the food—in class.

Gardening Share and Tell. Your child may want to show off her new knowledge of natural foods—through a classroom demonstration of sprouting.

Thanksgiving Project. For a school research project, your child can dig into the encyclopedia to find out exactly what the Pilgrims ate on that first Thanksgiving Day. Both you and your child might be surprised.

Have a Natural Foods Bake-off! You can organize a fun-filled bake-off through your PTA, church, or even the local natural foods store. Our Mrs. Gooch's Natural Foods Bake-off has always been fun and rewarding. Most of the recipes in Appendix B were a result of our early contests.

The rules for a natural foods bake-off are simple. All entrants must use only natural ingredients. No refined flour or sugar. No caffeine or cocoa. No artificial flavors, colors, preservatives, or harmful additives of any kind. No hydrogenated oils.

You can break the entries down into categories, too. Yeast Breads and Rolls. Main Dishes. Cookies. Cakes. Quick Breads and Muffins. Appetizers. Pies. ... etc.

You may want to give each entrant a natural foods conversion and substitution guide to help her convert her favorite recipe to an all-natural treat. You'll find our conversion guide in the recipe appendix.

Good luck! Have fun!

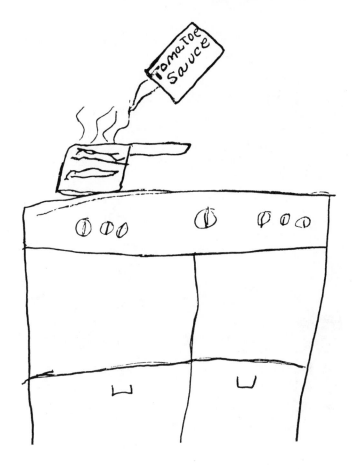

Macaroni

Boil water up to the top of the pan. Put in almost all of the macaroni.

You wait for a long time.

Buy a can of tomato sauce while you wait. Pour this on the macaroni.

I just don't know another thing you can do with it.

Terri Orloff

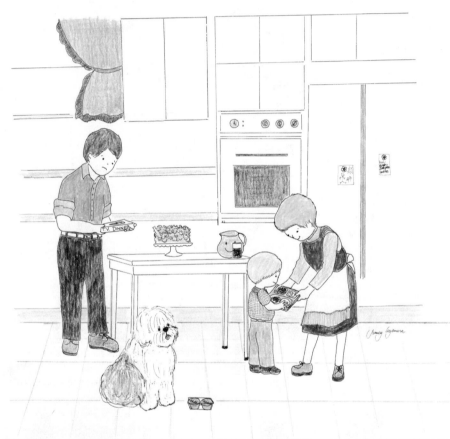

Is your Mate A Junk Food Junkie?

12

I remember a movie I saw in which a man and woman fell in love and got married. They were having a wonderful time together—until it became apparent that the man was an alcoholic. The woman tried her best to help him, but she wound up becoming an alcoholic herself. Then, as the story progressed, the man was able to control his alcoholism, but the woman was not. Tragically, after many verbal battles, they parted.

I tried to figure out why this tragic story came into my mind as I was sitting down to write this chapter. After some thought, I realized that when our mate doesn't share our feelings and attitudes about something as important as nutrition and health, the stage is set for a real War of Wills.

The purpose of this chapter is to help you avoid such a battle if your mate doesn't feel the same way about nutrition as you do. If your natural foods revolution turns into a battleground between you and your mate, there can be no winner. And the real loser will be your child.

This problem can rear its ugly head in almost as many forms as there are different types of relationships in our society. If you're still living with your first mate, the worst thing that can happen is your mate will be a junk food junkie who is totally unsympathetic to your goals and desires.

If you're divorced—as I am—then you may find yourself facing the problem on *two fronts at once*—at home with a new mate and away when your child is with his other parent! (I write this as a divorced mother who has her child living with her, but I am also aware that there are many children who live with their fathers.)

Before I get to my own story, I'd like to share the story of a good friend of mine, a man I'll call Tom. Tom and Darcy have a son named Josh. They're also divorced.

Tom is into natural foods. As a wholistic health practitioner, he knows that Josh needs to be on a natural foods diet in order to enjoy optimum health and reach his full potential.

Darcy does not understand, nor does she care to *try* to understand. When Josh is with her (which is most of the time), she feeds him TV dinners and junk food.

Tom is deeply saddened by this, but he is determined to do all he can to improve Josh's diet. Here are some of the things he does when Josh is with him on weekends: He grinds grains with his son and bakes whole grain goodies; he takes Josh shopping at the natural food store—where Josh gets to choose the items he'd like to eat; he takes Josh to the farm for fresh produce and eggs; they go on camping trips together; they bake bread, pies, and granola and make yogurt together; they team up on most of the activities mentioned in this book—in fact, Tom has been the *source* for many of the activities in this book!

Josh knows that when he's with his Daddy that there is going to be no deviation from the natural foods diet. No sugar, no refined flour, no junk food. And he accepts that.

He also knows that the time with Daddy is going to be extra-special and exciting, because Tom tries to make it so. Josh accepts the natural foods diet with no resistance—and proceeds to have a lot of fun whenever he's with his father.

Tom's main goal—because communication with Darcy seems to be impossible—is to teach Josh all he can. He is working, preparing, and educating for the day when Josh is old enough and mature enough to judge, decide, and speak for himself.

I include this story because I know there will be a lot of people out there who may be in a similar situation—one in which communication with the ex-spouse is going to be very difficult, if not impossible. I want you to know that there are others who share your problem. If there are no open doors of communication and sharing between you and your child's other parent, your best bet is to focus on your child—not with the intention of setting the child against the other parent, or confusing the child, but merely to give him as solid and true a natural foods experience as possible.

My situation with Kristin's father is not as desperate as Tom's is with Darcy. My ex-husband experienced natural foods in my household, but now he lives in a household where natural foods are not the rule. Although he was cooperative when we were together, he's cooperative in his present situation, too. So when Kristin goes over there, they don't often have the kind of pure, natural food I would like her to have.

I have handled this situation in many different ways, depending on the circumstances. Once, when Kristin was on a diet and wanted to take off five pounds, I pre-packaged all her food for the weekend, and she took it over to their house. She didn't make a big deal about it. She cooked all her own food for the entire weekend, and didn't make any special requirements for my ex-husband and his wife.

When she came back, Kristin felt really good. She had experienced responsibility, and—let me tell you—she received a lot of validation from me for taking care of herself so well. I congratulated her heartily on her success. She really *wanted* to do it the right way. I was quite proud of her, and let her know that.

To top it off, Kristin saw the fruits of her labors. When she got back, she found she had lost two pounds!

Of course, it's not always so easy. Every Sunday after church, Kristin's father and his new family go to a coffee shop for breakfast. It's a family affair and Kristin really enjoys it. At these times, she vacillates. Often, she will just have a hard-boiled egg, or cottage cheese, or a glass of orange juice. But there are other times when there is a big pile of sweet rolls on the table that she just can't resist.

Usually when this happens, Kristin will see and feel the results in her own body somewhere down the line. Her face will break out, or she'll notice she's gained some weight. She sees *for herself* the results of eating junk food.

There are other times when Kristin doesn't vacillate. She will help the family bake cakes right out of the cake mix boxes. Kristin enjoys the family experience of baking the cake, but she doesn't eat any of the cake after it's done.

I'm very glad we established natural foods as a family thing. Now, although Kristin's father's new family doesn't follow a natural foods diet, their caring for Kristin means that she is free to follow her dietary preferences as she sees fit. They don't make a big deal about it one way or the other. Kristin's father has seen the value of a natural foods diet, and to the extent of his ability, he has supported Kristin in her efforts to maintain her diet. Kristin's diet has not become a battleground between my ex-husband and me. Kristin comes out the winner every time.

I believe there are two worthy goals for a parent who finds his or her mate is (or *almost* is) a junk food junkie:

1. Don't make the child's diet a battleground between you and your spouse (or ex-spouse).

2. Strive to make your child the winner in all situations.

Don't Turn Your Child's Diet into a Food Fight!

I was fortunate. I had almost total sympathy and commitment from Kristin's father right from the start. Natural food was a family thing from the word go.

We're not all that lucky. I'm sure there are plenty of people out there who have heard one or more of the following.

"Oh, no. You're not getting *me* to eat that stuff!"

"What? Are we gonna have sprouts growing out of our mouths from now on?"

"Natural foods! But Purple Chemi-Doo-Dads *are* natural! It says so right here on the box! See, 'all natural ingredients!'"

"Does this mean I can't have my steak and potatoes anymore—and all we're gonna eat is beans and salads?"

"NO WAY!"

"You'll just have to cook two dinners, honey!"

When you approach a semi-sympathetic—or downright non-sympathetic—mate, be careful not to turn it into an "either-or" situation. Look back to Chapter 8—"Kids Eat The Darnedest Things." Well, *mates* eat the darnedest things, too. And if you approach your mate with the words: "No more of *this stuff* in the house," you're waving a red flag to start the food fight.

Everything I said in Chapter 8 applies to mates, too:

1. Don't try to change everything overnight.

2. Express the dietary change to natural foods in positive terms.

3. Let your mate know that the Old Favorites—or most of them, anyway—are still going to be there.

4. And don't just *say* they're going to be "better." *Make sure they're tastier and more fun to eat.*

My New Mate Was a Junk Food Junkie

I'll never forget the first time I had Harry over to my house for dinner. Harry was the Original Junk Food Junkie. As a child, he used to hide Sugar Sponge Cakes under his bed, so his sister and brother wouldn't find them. He once prided himself on his encyclopedic knowledge of the best burger joints and doughnut shops in the L.A. area! He even knew what times of the day each bakery pulled a fresh batch of doughnuts out of the oven!

Brother! Was Harry ever scared that when he came to my house he was going to have to sit down to a dinner of sprouts and raw vegetable juice—or some equally "weird" things.

Instead, what Harry found waiting for him on the dinner table were hamburgers (certified, naturally-grown, hormone and antibiotic-free)— a food with which he was quite familiar. He also found potato salad, and a raw vegetable salad. Everything was totally natural. The meat in the hamburgers was additive-free. The buns were whole wheat. The condiments and the dressing were sugar-free.

Needless to say, Harry was quite relieved. He really wanted to please me and try whatever I served him, but he didn't expect to find his favorite foods at my house. In his wildest dreams, he didn't imagine they'd taste as wonderful as they did!

Now ... Harry does much of the cooking—especially when we're entertaining, and it's all natural. Harry considers it an adventure as he learns more and more about the wonderful world of natural foods.

There's really no reason why you shouldn't be able to perform the same kind of magic with your mate. Good, natural foods are available that can meet and beat the best processed concoctions for both taste and value. You should be able to say to your mate: "You won't have to give up your hamburgers, spaghetti, lasagna, hot dogs, soda pop, crunchy breakfast cereal, bacon and eggs ... whatever!"

Of course, this is not to say you should limit your natural foods adventure to All-American favorites. You can use these foods as a good jumping off point into new and exciting natural flavors and recipes.

Make Sure Your Child Is Always the Winner

Really try your best to establish the change to natural foods as a family project. The more you share your goals and information with other members of the family, the more they will be ready to support those goals and help gather the information.

I know that it's a rare occurrence for both parents to happen upon some information and make up their minds to "go natural" at the same time. Usually, one or the other does some reading, some talking—and a revolution in thinking, feeling, and behavior begins. Do your best to share that revolution with your mate *right from the very first moment you are exposed to the new information*. Don't carry out your revolution in secret. If you share information and feelings with your mate right from the start, even if you don't get total sympathy or cooperation, or if your mate simply isn't interested, at least the changes won't come as complete surprises.

Nevertheless, you might still find yourself in a situation in which your mate says: "Why on earth are we doing that?" Or, "What in the world *for?*"

As you, I'm sure, are well aware by now, the entire process of changing to natural foods is an educational one. First, you educate yourself. Then, you educate your family. Then, as needed, you educate everyone your family is liable to come in contact with.

As with any educational process, it's most effective when taken *one step at a time*. My advice to "start early" applies to your mate as well as to your child. It applies to everyone you intend to educate. If you share your educational process with your mate and children right from the start, they will all learn right along with you. Your education in natural foods and health will belong to all of you. Isn't that the way you want it to be?

If you do happen to start later, and receive the "What on earth for?" response, you need to be armed with all the information and feelings and experiences that went into your own decision. Just as I advised you to share human feelings and experiences with your neighbors, you can do the same with that resistant mate.

Whether your resistant mate is your spouse or former spouse, the more communication that goes on, the better. You really can sit down with your mate and share your reasons for wanting your child's diet to be natural—and put it in the context of *this is really the best thing for the child.* Of course, you should be prepared to elaborate on *why* you feel it's best.

If the mate or parent is not willing to give natural foods a try in his or her own life, then you will have to sit down with your child and explain why this is so. Without making the other parent out to be a villain, simply say that "Daddy doesn't know how good natural foods can be right now—but maybe we can help show him as time goes on."

You also have the right—and the responsibility—to ask that there be some form of moderation when non-natural foods are made available. You can ask that especially offensive items not be used when the child is with the mate or other parent. You can also ask that the child's own wishes be respected when he wishes to refuse a certain food.

Don't Make the Other Mate the Villain

It's really important that you try very hard—no matter how uncooperative your mate is—not to make him or her out to be the villain, or the loser, or wrong. That puts pressure on the mate to prove he's right—and, likewise, prove that you're wrong. Then you have a battle of wills on your hands.

And on your child's hands, as well. Making the other mate out to be the villain puts pressure on your child. Children don't like to be put in the position of deciding which parent is right or wrong, which parent is the hero or the villain, which parent is the winner or the loser. Being in this position puts a lot of stress on a child—stress that the child really should not have to deal with at an early age—say before the age of seventy or eighty. It makes your child the loser, no matter who wins the battle between you and your mate.

Allow Your Child To Be the Winner—And The Teacher

Your child is the best person to tell your resistant mate about how good natural foods can be. All of the teaching principles and activities in this book can flow *from child to parent* just as effectively as from parent to child.

You can proceed with these assumptions in mind:

1. Your mate loves the child just as much as you do.
2. Your child loves his other parent just as much as he loves you.

If you operate under these assumptions, it puts your child in the middle, that's true. But it also gives you and your mate the opportunity to respond to your child's wishes, feelings, and needs. If your child can communicate to your mate that the desire for a natural foods diet comes *"from me"*, then there is nothing either you or your spouse can do but support that desire.

If your child can say to both of you, "If you love me, don't feed me junk!," then you can both do your best to make your child the winner.

Special Activities

You and your child can share all of the special activities in this book with your mate. The key to education is sharing. When you want to teach someone something, what you really want to do is share your knowledge with him. To get closer to the goal of enlisting the support of your mate, you can encourage your child to share all of his knowledge regarding natural foods—as well as all of the activities that have helped shape that knowledge—with his other parent.

Everyone likes to have someone they love *cook something* for them. If your child applies his new knowledge of natural foods to whip up something really special for your mate, and then presents it by saying: "I made this especially for you—and it's natural, because I love you!," is there a heart in even the most resistant parent that would not be softened *just a little bit?*

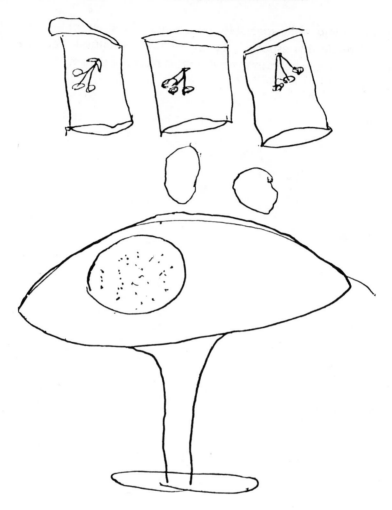

Cherry Pie

You need 5 cans of cherries. Put in 3 spoons of sugar, 4 spoons of milk and 2 eggs. Make a crust and put it *just* on top of the cherry stuff. Put it in the oven for 5 minutes.

Take it out, and while it cools my Mom can clean up.

Loren Lovgren

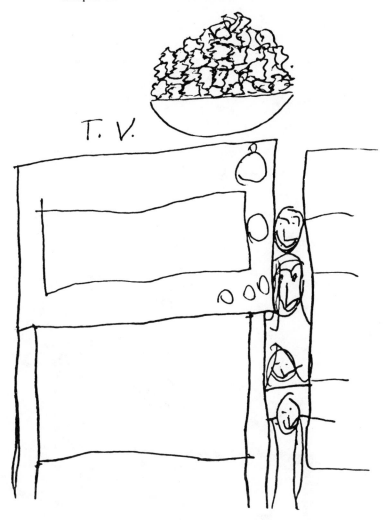

Pop Corn

Put 3 scoops of Crisco in a popper. Put in 1 scoop of popcorn.

Take a knife and slice 3 scoops of butter and put it in a low oven.

The pop corn stops popping. Put it in a bowl. Pour the sauce on and put all the salt on the pop corn and that's all!

Jon Washizaki

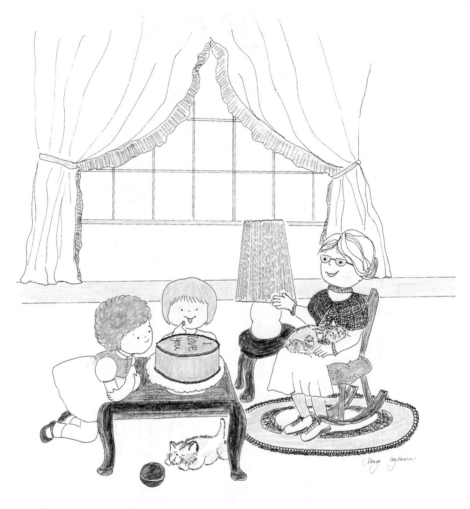

When In-laws Show Love
With Outlaw Food

13

Somewhere back in the Dark Ages, the candy manufacturers made a secret pact with Grandmas and Grandpas. The terms of the pact were that Grandmas and Grandpas would always show their love for their grandchildren by giving them candy.

In return, the grandparents were told they would never, ever, have to accompany their grandchildren to the dentist's office. It was left to the parents to stand by and hold their children's hands while the dentist drilled away the cavities left by the candy.

The candy manufacturers kept up their end of the bargain by making more gargantuan Easter baskets every year—layer after layer of candy eggs and chocolate bunnies hidden in the plastic grass, wrapped in yards of gaily colored cellophane. Who could resist the temptation of tearing through that cellophane and finding all the sweet treasure?

What parents would even think of denying their children all that fun? After all, "Easter comes only once a year ... ."

But so does Christmas—and on Christmas, Grandma brings dozen after dozen of her sugar cookies—the same ones she's made for decades, the ones with all the multicolored, glassy sugar sparkles on them.

And the Fourth of July comes only once a year—when Grandpa barbecues pound after pound of nitrate-laden hot dogs.

And so does Thanksgiving—when we give thanks that Grandma makes only one or two sugary pies since she's saving her energy for Christmas.

And each of the birthdays come only once a year ... along with all the cake and ice cream ... .

And then there are all the other times when Grandma and Grandpa—and hosts of other relatives—get to show how much they love your children by giving them junk food.

We keep running into a simple fact of life. In our culture, we show how much we love each other through gifts of food. I'm sure this practice harkens back to a time long before that dark day when the candy manufacturers made their pact with grandparents, back to a time when food was scarce and sharing food was sharing survival as well as love.

This instinct we have to give food to loved ones runs so deep that it would be difficult, if not impossible, to ignore, deny, or obliterate it. And as I've said before, my aim in this book is *not* to suggest that you should stop showing love through food.

On the contrary, since I believe that food is—and should be—closely bound with feelings of love, it is all the more important that we give our loved ones the best food we can.

You know this, and I know this. Now, if someone would only tell Grandma and Grandpa and Auntie and Uncle and all the rest!

That responsibility—as if you didn't know—rests on your shoulders. But take heart. It can be done. If you've come this far—if you've managed to get the junk out of your diet, out of your cupboard, out of your mate's diet, out of your child's school, and have neutralized the effects of the TV hucksters—you'll probably find that dealing with in-laws who give your child outlaw food will be among the easier tasks in your crusade.

"Hold it right there, Sandy! Are you trying to tell me that it will be easier for me to talk _____ (substitute your favorite name for your in-law) into dumping the junk than it was to talk the entire school system into serving bean sprouts and veggieburgers? You sure don't know _____!"

You're right, I don't know all the _____s out there, but I do know one thing about grandparents. Their love for their grandchildren is the most splendidly *unconditional* love your children will find anywhere. Grandparents are so thrilled with their grandchildren that they grant unconditional acceptance without a struggle. That's why grandparents are always accused of "spoiling" their grandchildren.

The trick is to get them to "spoil" your child without spoiling his diet. To do that, you have to educate them. There's a message you want them to get, and that message is: If you love them, don't feed them junk!

You *can* take the "sneaky" approach—actually, a variation of the sneaky approach. Instead of sneaking good food into your family's diet, you sneak the bad food out of it. In other words, when Grandma shows up with the brownies, smile and put them on the counter—and then in the trash as soon as she's out the door.

I don't feel any better about this approach than I do about the other manifestations of the sneaky approach. By taking the undercover approach to the problem, no one grows or learns anything worthwhile. And in this particular case, two additional things happen that you may not want to happen.

First, your child will learn that the best way to deal with problems concerning other people is through deception. There's no way you can avoid teaching this lesson if you choose to secretly dump Grandma's junk food gifts. The child is going to receive the gift from Grandma—and then want to know where it went. Are you going to compound the lie?

The second unfortunate side effect of secretly "disappearing" outlaw food is that it blocks the love that Grandma sincerely meant to deliver through the food. (Note: I understand that there will be occasions when dumping the junk will be the only available course of action—such as when in-laws simply refuse to cooperate. I will deal with those circumstances below.)

Isn't it better that the love that flows so unconditionally from Grandma and Grandpa be allowed to reach your child—in the form of good food, or some other acceptable gift?

I think it is. If you think so, too, your first order of business is to communicate that fact to Grandma and Grandpa, along with some other very pertinent facts. Basically, you can take the same approach as you did with other potentially resistant people, such as teachers, neighbors, and mates: Communicate. Ask for help. Share.

As with teachers, neighbors, and mates, your communication will be more effective if it is on a human level: "Mom, this is what's going on in our diets. We've learned some rather interesting things, and we're doing our best to eat all natural foods. We're trying very hard, and we're really feeling a lot better. Johnnie hasn't had a cold for three months, and you remember how sick he used to be all the time ... .

"Now, we just started a few months ago. But Susie across the street started over a year ago and her children have been feeling so much better ... .

"Mom and Dad, we know you love Johnnie very much and that you want to show your love, and *we really need your help in this* ... ."

The best way to enlist someone's support is to get them involved as much as possible. If you've been doing your homework, you've been substituting your child's favorite "junky" foods with natural treats and goodies. You should have some idea of what his real favorites are. Well, let Grandma, Grandpa, and all the Aunties and Uncles who love to bake know, too. Share the recipes with them.

"Mom and Dad, I know you always show your love by bringing something for Johnnie. That's so sweet of you, but when you come next time, could you bring some kind of natural treat? Let me give you some examples of things he really likes."

You can even go so far as to devise substitute recipes for the very goodies Grandma usually brings—and then share them with her. Or, you might ask Grandma to share the recipe with you, and then go about devising a substitute.

You can also try getting Grandma and Grandpa to show their love in some way not connected with food. Tell them about something your child has been wanting for a long time:

"Johnnie has been wanting a baseball for such a long time, Dad. He'd probably love that more than six dozen chocolate chip cookies ... ."

Or ... "Johnnie really needs a new raincoat ... or a pair of boots ... or a new backpack ... and he'd really appreciate it and think of you every time he used it—whereas those sugar cakes you made will be gone and forgotten sooner than you can imagine ... ."

You can try this approach. I believe you will succeed in getting Grandma and Grandpa to buy that baseball or pair of boots or new coat or whatever. But if I know grandparents, your child is also going to get the cookies and cake thrown in for good measure—unless you are sure to communicate your new standards for food.

There's really no way to solve this problem without making a stand. Sooner or later, you're going to have to sit down with Grandma and Grandpa and make it clear that you do not want your child eating certain food. As with other people, you will be more effective if you share and communicate on a human level—without preaching.

"Grandma, please stop murdering Johnnie with those damn brownies!" is not going to work anywhere near as well as "Grandma, you know, I'll just bet Johnnie would love it even more if you made your brownies with carob, honey, whole wheat flour, and peanut butter."

Another line that probably won't be too effective is: "Mom and Dad, you've got to stop eating all that junk! You're killing yourselves! Really, the best diet for you is ... ."

Whole books could be written about how to change your parents and in-laws' diets to natural foods. I'm going to pass on that right now, and you should, too. My purpose in this book is to tell you how to effectively change your child's diet—and make it stick. Besides, I'm sure that if you set out to convert everyone from Grandma to the mailman, you would not be as effective *at home with your child.*

Most grandparents will understand and respond to your sincere call for help. After all, if you make them understand that the best way to show love to your child is no longer through junk food but through wholesome natural food, what else can they do but jump on the bandwagon and cooperate ... ?

"What do you mean, calling my sugar-fat doughnuts 'junk food?' They certainly didn't hurt you any, did they? And I baked them for you every week when you were Johnnie's age!"

Or ... as I've heard many times in a radio interview when the interviewer "goes to the phones" for listeners' comments, an old timer will call in and say something like "What's this nonsense about junk food being harmful? I've been eating this way all my life and I'm seventy-five!"

My answer to that statement is always a respectful "No, you really haven't been eating 'that way' for all your life. You did not eat the kind of junk that's available today when you were a child. In the last twenty years or so, the amount of artificial chemicals, refined sugar, and other potentially harmful additives in food has increased astronomically. You were not exposed to anywhere near as much junk when you were young. You grew up on good, wholesome, natural foods, and I want my child to grow up on them, too."

On the radio, my response usually does the trick—meaning the older person will respond with an "A-hah! Hmmm ... I'm beginning to see your point ... . I understand what you mean, now."

All you're really asking is that your child have the opportunity to grow up on the same wholesome food that his grandparents did. Communicate to Grandma and Grandpa that you're not trying to "improve

upon them," that all you want is to get back to an integrity they enjoyed when they were growing up.

It was, of course, a different story when *we* were growing up.
Those "sugar-fat doughnuts" that Mom made for us, which we gob-
bled up along with all the love that came with them, present your
toughest challenge in dealing with Grandma and Grandpa. You might
try a variation of my answer to the old timers who call in on my radio
shows.

"Mom, it's true that I literally lived on your sugar-fat doughnuts and
brownies and chocolate chip cookies when I was a kid ... but I am concerned that *I* may not be as healthy and strong as you, and I really want
Johnnie to have as wholesome a natural foods diet as possible ...
Besides, we didn't understand then how foods like that can affect us.
Now, our understanding has grown. Besides, I want Johnnie to be
even healthier than I am—and healthier than you are, too."

Don't Be Afraid To Make a Stand

In-laws—whether they're yours or your mate's— have a way of
being particularly stubborn about some things. Communicating, sharing, and asking for help and support may win you nods of the head
and smiles—but when they walk in the door, the doughnuts and the
brownies and the chocolate cakes and the sugar cookies may still come
with them.

You have the right, and the responsibility, to be firm. If you've
touched all the bases, and the in-laws still show their love with junk, it's
time to start dumping the junk or sending it back. In either case, I don't
think it's a good idea to be sneaky. Tell Grandma exactly what you're
doing with her brownies—and tell her why. Hope that she gets the
message.

If your child will be visiting Grandma's house for an extended time,
you have a special problem. Your child may be at the mercy of Grandma's unresponsiveness to your dietary standards. I believe you can be
firm in this circumstance as well. You can refuse to allow your child to
spend that much time there if your requests to dump the junk are not
respected.

I believe that a course of action this drastic should only be used as a
last resort. I also believe, however, that it will work. There should not

be any barriers between a child and his grandparents, and it's your job to make unresponsive in-laws understand that *they* are putting up the barriers by not respecting your dietary standards for your child. Also make them understand that they can *bring the barriers down* by participating in your and your child's natural foods revolution.

Your Child Can Be the Teacher

I want to share with you a letter I received from a Brownie troop leader after I led her troop on a tour of one of my markets:

Dear Mrs. Gooch,

From all the girls and leaders of Brownie troop 214, a huge 'Thank you.' Our tour of your store was fascinating and may influence our girls for the rest of their lives. They truly took to heart your personal story.

An example of this took place in our home during Christmas. My daughter, Angela, retold your story and described your store to her grandparents. They listened with the skeptical attitude of being 'too old' for changes in lifestyle. However, Angela kept after them for the rest of their visit with 'no salt, cut the fat off your meat, use brown bread,' etc. At times I wanted to put a muzzle on her! But I felt happy that she was going to be aware of these things.

We saved all the food you gave us and built our last meeting around healthful snacking. It was a feast!

Again, many thanks for your hospitality and generosity.

This letter demonstrates that the best person to level with Grandma and Grandpa is Grand-kid, himself. Again, once you've come this far in the process, you've not only been teaching your child about food, but also about how to handle situations in which people are offering him food that's not good for him. He can handle Grandma and Grandpa the same way—with a little more diplomacy and love, of course.

Explain to your child that his grandparents love him very much and that they are showing their love by giving him this food ... "but they just don't know as much about nutrition and what's good for us as we do—so we'll have to help them learn."

There is a difference between your telling your in-laws or your parents that junk food is not good for *them* and your child's telling them that junk food is not good for *him*. Exploit that difference to the fullest, because it's really your strongest point. It's one thing for Grandma and Grandpa to ignore your pleading about chemical additives and sugar and the rest.

But how can they do anything but respond when the object of all their love says, "Grandma and Grandpa, I'm happy that you love me so very much ... but I really don't like those sugary doughnuts and those chocolate things and that candy. I would rather have these natural goodies ... "?

It may take years for your in-laws or parents to come around to heeding your dietary laws, but if your child has it together enough to lay down the law himself, they'll get the message in a matter of minutes. They may laugh and say, "How cute!" (if your child is young)—but you can be sure they'll get the message and do their best to make the child happy as soon as they can.

I've seen it happen too many times—on the most stubborn Grandparents—to believe otherwise: "If you want to spoil me, Grandma and Grandpa ... I know a better way."

Special Activities

Turn the tables on Grandma and Grandpa. Have your child select some of his favorite natural goodies. Help him prepare them, and then bring them along when you visit Grandma and Grandpa.

"Hey, Grandma, you're always bringing me goodies when you visit. I thought I'd bake something for you for a change! I made this batch of cookies (or whatever)! I love you, Grandma!"

Write a book! Start by helping your child make a list of his favorite foods. Then have him draw colorful pictures of each one, as well as pictures showing his improved health and vitality. You can help him write down the recipes, and then combine all of this material in a booklet titled *If You Love Me, Don't Feed Me Junk!* The booklet can serve as a gift for Grandmas, Grandpas, Aunties, and Uncles.

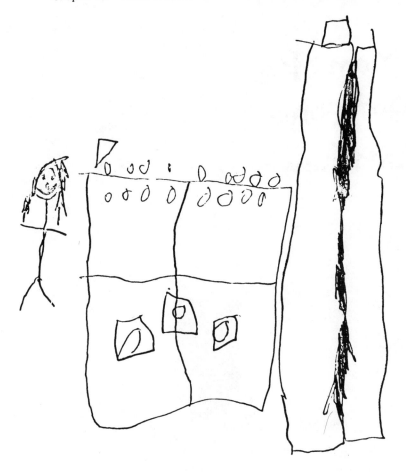

A Grandma Picnic

Put tortillas in the oven. Cook 6 pounds of meat on the Bar-b-q. Take out the tortillas. Now put the potatoes on the bar-b-q. Now we're gonna roast the marshmallows. Then my Mom cooks some Jello and custard pie.

Jump in the car and pick up Grandma. (She lives in Las Vegas so this will take awhile.) When we get back, Grandma will want to eat so we'll all go outside and start our picnic.

Shawn McAnich

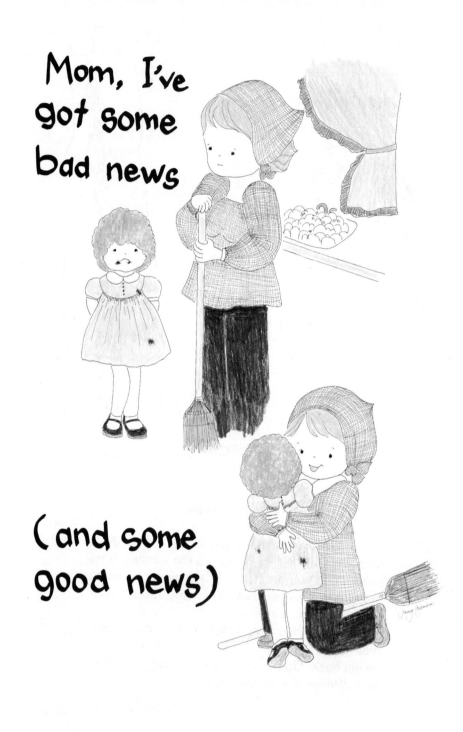

14

My friend Barbara's six year old, Cindy, is absolutely the cutest little thing you ever saw. She has curly ringlets of red hair that hang down over her forehead, freckles here, there, and everywhere—depending on the time of year—and sparkling blue eyes that just never quit smiling at you.

Barbara told me that one day Cindy rushed in from playing outside with a friend and stood before her, hands knit nervously behind her back, with the tell-tale signs of a devoured chocolate bar smudged around her pouting little lips.

"Mommie ... I did a bad thing ... I ... ate a candy bar at Jackie's house."

Barbara looked down at her daughter, who stands about three-feet tall but who has a way of looking so-o-o small and vulnerable ... Barbara felt her heart and mind race. This was a plot! A conspiracy by Jackie and her mother to undermine her parental authority! There go all those months of patient teaching and artwork and cleaning up the kitchen after she and Cindy made a royal mess "learning how to bake natural goodies."

Then Barbara saw those sparking blue eyes ... and those smudges ... and those pudgy little hands knitting so-o-o nervously behind Cindy's back ... .

And she remembered how good chocolate bars looked to her when she was six years old ... how good they still looked!

And Barbara laughed, knelt down, and gave Cindy the biggest hug she'd given her little girl in days!

"Thank you, Cinderella!" Barbara said, "Mommie is so glad that you came right home and told me."

Children are really great. They're so ... passionate about everything. Have you ever known a child to be halfway about anything? You'll rarely hear a child say, "Well, Mom, there were some good points and some not-so-good points about that ... ."

Instead, you'll hear:

"I hate that spinach!"

"I love that cake you made, Mom!"

"I want that, Mom. I've just gotta have it!"

"Ycchh! No way! I don't want it! No-o-o!"

Children are more up front and straightforward than adults. They haven't yet learned to follow all the mental detours we go through before we do something. We adults generally have to talk ourselves into or out of something before we make up our minds—unless, of course, we're in such an emotionally volatile state—anger, sadness, love, or whatever—that we simply "don't think before we act."

Children are *always* that volatile, bless them. The younger they are, the more in touch with their appetites and feelings they will be—and the less in touch with rationalized diversions. As they grow older, the rationalizations will gain more and more in strength—though we hope that they will *always* be in touch with their feelings. I believe that a worthy goal for the overall education of a child is to encourage her to stay in touch with her feelings while learning those pathways of reason that will enable her to be a more effective and fulfilled adult.

We don't want to discourage her from acting in accordance with her feelings, because it's her feelings that will tell her that natural foods are better. She will understand that natural food *tastes better* and that she *feels better* when she eats natural food and avoids junk.

It takes time for this to happen. It takes time for a child to learn, for everything we teach her to sink in. Along the way, there may be occasions when those tell-tale chocolate smudges appear around those little pouting lips. Isn't it better to treat these incidents as part of the learning process rather than as rebellious deviations from it or conspiracies to undermine it? Doesn't Barbara's response to Cindy's chocolate bar look like a lot more fun than the alternative scenario?

"My God, Cindy! A candy bar! What's the matter with you, huh? How many times have I told you? Well, Miss Candy Bar, no dessert for you tonight, and I'm baking your favorite, too!"

Mistakes Are Part of the Learning Process

Naturally, there's a lot more to handling your child's mistakes than smiling and giving an affectionate hug. But Barbara's acceptance of her daughter—the smile and the hug—was the best "first aid" for Cindy's mistake. After all, Cindy may have made a mistake in eating the candy bar, but that was a "crime of passion," which she freely acknowledged. Barbara's smile and hug were not rewards for the crime, but rewards for Cindy's demonstration that she had already begun to build and follow the exact same rational pathways Barbara had been teaching her.

Barbara understood that we do not want to weaken or discourage that wonderful connection a child has with her feelings. Rather, as adults accustomed to taking all those rationalized detours, we need to learn to take some of those shortcuts ourselves—in order to better understand our child, what she's feeling, and why she acted a certain way.

Barbara had good reason to reward her daughter and even to rejoice over the good news her daughter had brought her. When a child admits a mistake to you, her honesty presents you with opportunities that reach far beyond teaching her anything about nutrition. It means that she feels close enough to you, free enough, to share some very powerful information about herself and her life.

What are you going to do with this opportunity? This is your big chance to practice our six principles in Chapter 3, "Teaching Is An Act Of Love," *under fire.*

Love Unconditionally

Don't allow a little thing like a candy bar or a Purple Chemi-Doo-Dad to get in the way of your love and acceptance for your child. Don't let her mistake block the communication between you. Remember that her deepest need is to believe that she is lovable and valuable and acceptable just by virture of *being*.

Love unconditionally. Accept unconditionally. Don't try to motivate her by switching your love and acceptance on and off. If you use your love as a carrot on the end of a stick in front of her, you will ultimately succeed only in damaging her and your relationship.

To have to perform for love creates anxiety, doubt, and resentment. These emotions are the enemies of love. No lessons or standards—whether dietary or otherwise—are worth damaging the love between you and your child.

Mirror Your Child's Feelings

If you don't want your child to be afraid of your feelings and value judgments about her behavior, then you shouldn't be afraid of her feelings, either. You shouldn't be afraid to try to empathize with her, mirror her feelings, reach down deep into yourself, and try to duplicate those feelings in yourself.

When your child makes a mistake or has a hard time giving up a particular food, you want to be able to let her know that you know how it feels to be in that situation. You want to be able to give her something of yourself—your experience and feeling.

"Gee, Cindy ... I know how it feels to have someone offer you something and really want to take it ... ."

"Gee, I'll bet you thought that candy bar would just be the greatest thing to eat! I know how that is. I've felt that way about lots of things I wanted."

"Yes ... I know how hard it is when you're at a birthday party and there are twelve other kids there. I can understand what you went through. I've been on diets before—and then slipped off, so I can really understand the decision you made to have the cake ... and the ice cream ... and the cookies ... and the Purple Chemi-Doo-Dads. Maybe next time you'll be able to say no."

Let her know that you make mistakes, too—and that you try your best to learn from them. You do the wrong things from time to time, but you really want to do better. One of the most important messages a parent can send to a child—and vice versa—is the message of shared understanding.

"Cindy, I know how it feels to make a mistake. I've made some real whoppers, and I've felt totally worthless—like I would *never* be able to do the right thing. But you know, I always found that I could learn to do better. And I know that you will, too."

How Does Your Child Feel About It?

Allow your child to share with you her own feelings about what happened—as much as she wants to share, that is. Once you've let her know that you do understand how hard it is to always do the right thing, you can delve a bit deeper into the particular circumstances that led up to this mistake.

"How did you get roped into that?"

"How do you feel about it now?"

"What made you decide to go ahead and have the candy bar?"

"Was it a good experience? Did you enjoy it?"

There are two very good reasons why you may want to delve deeper into your child's feelings about what has been a difficult situation for her. Often, a child will sense the effect the junk food is having on her body. If you can help her focus her consciousness on *how she really feels* rather than on fear and defensiveness, she will be that much more ahead of the game in building those pathways between thought, feeling, and action. She will be closer to being able to connect her genuine knowledge of how the junk food will make her feel with whether or not she really wants it—and whether she's going to have it. The second reason for digging a little deeper into what led up to the mistake is that she may be operating on misunderstood information, which you need to know about before you can correct.

"Thank you for telling me about the chocolate-coated rice cakes you ate. I really appreciate your honesty. But ... I'm a little curious as to why you ate them?"

"Well, gee, Mom ... we have rice cakes all the time!"

"Yes we do ... but not chocolate-coated ones."

"Well ... we have these here. They're coated."

"Yes, but that's a carob coating. I know they look almost exactly alike, but carob is quite a bit different from chocolate. Let me explain the difference ... ."

You Can Be Honest, Too

I don't mean to give the impression that you shouldn't share your feelings with your child, too. This is not a competition to see who can be the most laid-back, easy-going parent. It's much better to say what you're actually feeling, rather than trying to hide it. It's better to tell your child, "I am angry that you ate that box of chocolate chip cookies and drank the six-pack of cola."

Your feelings will not remain hidden, believe me. Isn't it better that you share them verbally, rather than in some other way? Feelings like anger and resentment have a way of building and growing stronger if we don't acknowledge them, if we shove them back down and pretend they're not there.

If you have strong feelings about your child's mistake, by all means share them, too. Just be careful that you do not trample your child's self-esteem in the process. Share your feelings of anger without pulling back your acceptance and love.

"Gee, I don't feel too good about what you did. I feel angry. We've worked hard—both of us—to learn all about good food and what junk food can do to us. It makes me feel angry right now that you ate junk food, and I want you to know that. But I also want you to know that I feel very good that you've told me about it, and I have confidence in you. I know how you felt—and I also know that you'll try even harder next time—and succeed."

Don't Let the Error Slip By

Acknowledge the error as an error, and also make sure your child does the same. Don't allow the mistake to get by without its being seen as a deviation from a planned course of behavior agreed upon by you and your child. The mistake is part of the process of learning, so put it solidly inside of the context of whatever positive lesson you want to reinforce.

As I said at the beginning of this chapter, it does take time for lessons to sink in. Time and repetition are the key, and this mistake is a golden opportunity to repeat the lesson.

Affirm the Positive

Positive affirmation provides a structure for dealing with mistakes and fitting them into the context of learning rather than regretting. You can affirm the positive by saying to your child:

"You usually are quite good about choosing your food, and I know you want to take good care of yourself."

Call attention to her previous accomplishments. Let her know you are confident she will have even greater success and satisfaction in the future.

When you talk about the future—whether you're giving instructions or repeating a previous lesson—don't affirm the negative by calling attention to the possibility that the mistake will be repeated.

"If you eat any more candy bars, I'll have to eliminate your dessert for a month!"

Remember that by focusing your attention on the possiblity, you are giving it more energy. Besides, it's always more effective to promise a reward if the instructions are carried out than to promise punishment if they're not. Call attention to the health benefits of good food more often than you express the dangers of junk food. You want your child to keep positive goals in mind rather than anxiety-producing thoughts of being pursued by failure.

Positive affirmation also helps support honesty. If your child knows you are more interested in growth and improvement—and not so much in punishment—if she knows you will respond to mistakes by affirming positive values and actions, she'll feel free to be honest.

She should, at all times, feel and believe that you are more interested in knowing the truth than in maintaining an ideal or status quo. To achieve this, you must never punish her or withdraw your acceptance when she tells you about something you would prefer she had not done.

It will be easier for her to be honest if she knows you will not attack her point of view. Let her know that you appreciate, respect, and really want to know what she sees, feels, and believes. Her point of view may be quite different from yours. Nevertheless, allow her the freedom to develop her own point of view by not vigorously challenging her when hers differs from yours. Even when you feel strongly that there is a mistake around the corner, let her see—or even make—the mistake. Then, let her be free to tell you about it.

Don't "make points" at her expense by saying, "I told you so ... " or, "I knew that would happen." These statements are attacks on her vulnerable self-esteem.

Instead, support her ever-developing point of view by putting mistakes in the proper perspective. Mistakes are to be learned from and acknowledged, but not to be worn around the neck like badges of self-scorn.

Keep those lines of communication between you and your child uncluttered by past errors. Keep them open and free. You will both need them.

My daughter Kristin knows she is free to make her own decisions regarding food. She knows what foods I believe are best, and she knows that I expect her to choose the best food for herself, too. But she also knows that she is free to be uncompromisingly honest in telling me about what foods she eats outside our home. If she has a doughnut or a soft drink, she can tell me.

I don't punish her. She doesn't have to make up any remedial "points"—and never has had to. I know she has learned her lesson well enough. She has learned that she can communicate with me. She has learned she is free to make her own choices. And, most importantly, she has learned she can be honest about the consequences *not only to me but to herself.*

Occasionally, Kristin will say, "I had half a doughnut at school today, and I don't really believe I enjoyed it that much. I felt too full all day. I'm going to try harder to avoid that stuff."

Kristin always comes back to what she has a feel for, what she knows is best for her. She makes her choices with reference to herself—not because I, or anybody else, wants her to.

Special Actitivies

Attitude is all-important in choosing activities after your child has gone on a junk food binge. I believe it's important to do two things:

1. Avoid imparting the feeling that the activity is a remedial one, like writing "I will not eat candy bars" across the blackboard four million times.

2. Give the child a good experience with natural foods *as soon as possible*.

By now, you may know your child's favorite special activity from this book. Maybe it's baking bread, carob brownies, or oatmeal cookies. Maybe she'd enjoy a trip to the farm or to the natural foods bakery. It's a good idea to do something that reinforces your mutual commitment to natural foods.

Don't worry about this activity being interpreted as a reward. So what if it is, anyway? After all, your child's honesty and awareness deserve to be rewarded, don't they?

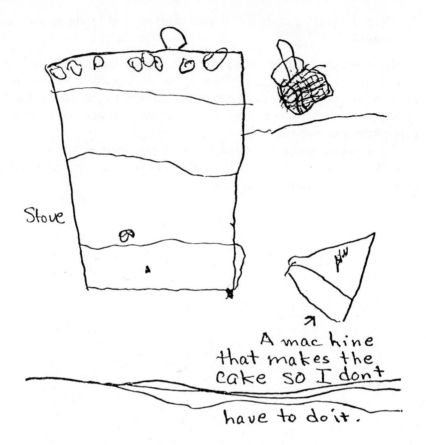

Stove

A machine
that makes the
cake so I don't
have to do it.

Cake

First, you go to the store and buy chocolate, frosting and cream. Then, you come home.

Here's the start. First, you put the cream in a pile. Then, put the frosting in a pile, and then the chocolate in a pile. Mix the 3 piles in a mixer. Put this in the oven at 3,000°. Take it out and put it in the refrigerator to make it cold again. Then, take it out and mix it up. Then, put it back in the oven at 5,000°.

This sure is a different way to make a cake!

Danny Ross

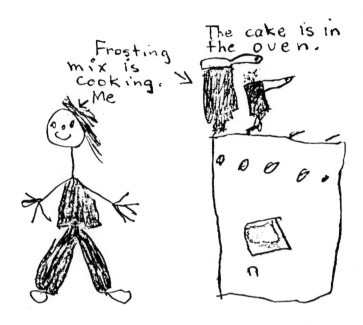

Frosting mix is cooking.

Me

The cake is in the oven.

Chocolate Cake

You need butter all over two pans. Put flour on top of the butter. Any flour left over, you dump in the sink. Open up a package of cake mix and dump it in a bowl. Put in 1 egg and ½ cup of water. Mix up all the ingredients. Pour this in the two pans for 25 minutes. Put it in a 100° oven and if it is not done, you cook it for 15 minutes more.

For the frosting, you use another mix. Just dump in eggs and mix it up.

Clyde Yokoi

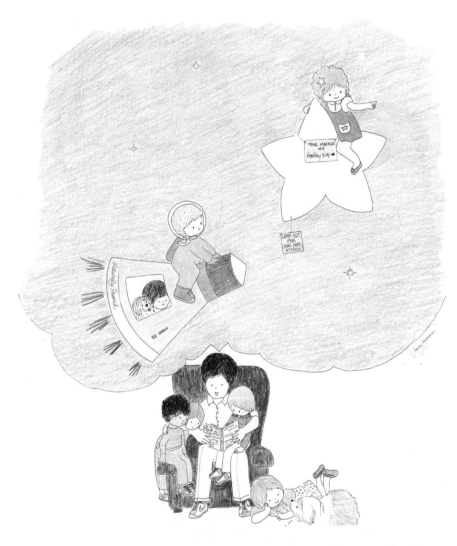

Is your child special?

15

I can see the letter now, at the top of a good-sized stack:

"Sandy, we're going absolutely nuts here! What kind of mess have you gotten us into? We dumped all the junk out of our cupboards, spent two whole days at the natural foods store replacing all the junk with what you call wholesome natural foods, and now we're miserable! We've never felt worse in our lives! We have headaches, we're tired, we feel sick most of the time—and we haven't touched a molecule of junk food in more than a week! What's happening to us?"

And then the letter below that one:

"Sandy, HELP! Little Timmy has been just wonderful. I did everything you said, and Timmy and his Dad have responded really well—except for one little problem that's driving me up the wall! They gave up their Sugar Bunnies for breakfast, their Fast Food Greaseburgers for lunch, and the Purple Chemi-Doo-Dads for snacks. But Timmy will simply not give up his chocolate. He *cries* for it! He wakes up sniffling in the middle of the night and wants a chocolate bar or a cup of hot chocolate to get to sleep! He's been so good in giving up all the other junk, I just don't know what to do. What's going on?"

---

*My special thanks to Los Angeles nutritionist Joyce Virtue for all her generous help in preparing this chapter.

169

My answer to both these letters is the same. What's going on is an allergy-addiction withdrawal. Your bodies—and the bodies of your children—have been adjusting to the junk, or the foods you're really allergic to, for a long, long time. Our bodies are so wonderful at adjusting that you hardly even noticed what the foods were doing to you and your children.

Then along comes Sandy Gooch, who tells you to dump the junk and eat natural foods. You take her advice, dump the junk, and start eating natural foods.

Bingo! No more sugar highs! No more toxins coming in to stimulate the system! No more of those additives, those glorious chemicals that gave your immune system a real run for its money for so long.

But wait a minute ... the body is confused. It had gotten so used to that constant assault, that it now actually *craves* the excitement of the battle. "Let them at me," it cries, with headaches and fatigue. "I'm bored! I want some *action!*"

I know all about how devastating and insidious food allergies can be. Remember, my own natural foods revolution began with an allergy that almost ended my life.

I planned this chapter to help parents whose children might be susceptible to one or more allergies to foods or to other substances found in our food supply. The more I investigated the rapidly growing subject of allergies and food sensitivities, the more I found additional reasons why this chapter was even more important than I had originally planned.

Here is what I learned:

1. Food allergies and sensitivities are more widespread and insidious than we commonly believe.

2. Many people—children especially—are allergic to common foods and food additives.

3. People—especially children—are quite often *addicted* to the very foods they're most allergic to!

4. When we withdraw from foods we're allergic—or addicted—to, we can experience withdrawal symptoms ranging from mild discomfort to severe physical and emotional disruptions.

5. These withdrawal symptoms can complicate, interfere with, and generally sabotage a family's switch to natural foods.

6. There is a relatively simple, moderately expensive ($200-300), medical test that can determine food allergies and sensitivities.

7. There is a slightly more complicated, though free, do-it-yourself at-home method of determining food allergies and sensitivities.

8. The very same principles and strategies that apply to families without allergies also apply to families with allergies.

9. I also learned, from veterinarian Alfred Jay Plechner, D.V.M., of the California Animal Hospital, 1736 South Sepulveda Blvd., Los Angeles, Calif, 90025, that all of the above points can also apply to *animals!* Dr. Plechner has treated hundreds of animals for nutritional problems, food sensitivities and allergies that have caused such symptoms as itchy, flaky skin; upset stomach; vomiting; enteritis; epilepsy; behavioral abnormalities; urinary tract diseases; and other common disorders in pets.)

Withdrawal Symptoms May Sabotage You

If you have been following my suggestions throughout this book—and you're still having trouble getting your child to give up certain foods, especially sugary, additive-laden junk foods—you can suspect an allergy addiction. Your child's physiological tie to the food may be so strong that he cannot give it up—even though he is actually allergic or sensitive to the food.

My advice is to *keep at it*. Withdrawal symptoms, which may even mimic the symptoms of the allergy itself, often surface when a family changes to natural foods. If you stick to the natural foods diet, your child's (as well as your family's) health and well-being will eventually improve.

It will take time. During that time, you and your children may be extra-sensitive to the allergenic foods. If you remember my story, when I was coming out of my illness by changing my diet to natural foods, there were several times when the least little slip would put me back in the hospital!

You may have extra-strong cravings for some of the foods you've given up. *Don't let these cravings sabotage your natural foods diet.* Now that you are aware of what's actually taking place—that your body is adjusting to the new situation—you can wait out the storm of withdrawal symptoms.

How Allergies and Food Sensitivities Develop

There once was a time when foods were truly seasonal. That meant if a food wasn't in season, people simply didn't have any of it. It also meant that when a food was in season, people could get all they wanted—and usually did. Food allergies and sensitivities were rare.

Today, thanks to modern agribusiness and rapid transportation, we have access to an incredible variety of foods all year round. We can have as much as we want, any day of the year. We also have access— through our food—to many chemicals that people never before even imagined existed, let alone ate. Food allergies and sensitivities are widespread.

What does availability have to do with allergy? Plenty. It's a rule of thumb that *we develop allergies and sensitivities to foods that we overuse.* The reason for this isn't difficult to explain. Our bodies require enzymes to properly digest and metabolize our foods. Because of biochemical individuality, we don't all have the same ability to manufacture these enzymes. If our supply of metabolic enzymes necessary to digest a particular food runs out, the body has a tough time handling the food. The food may be treated as if it were an invading, toxic substance, and an unpleasant reaction may occur.

With a food allergy, that reaction can be immediate and violent. With a food sensitivity, the reaction may take hours—or even days—to take full effect.

If we consume a particular food once in a great while, our enzyme supply can usually replenish itself. If we consume that food day after day for weeks, months, and years, the chances are good that our enzyme supply might be in a perpetual state of depletion. In that case, the food would always provoke some kind of toxic reaction in the body— an allergic response.

When foods were available only in season, most of them weren't around long enough for sensitivities or enzyme deficiencies to develop. Some foods, of course, were stored or were available all year—foods such as wheat, corn, and milk. It's no coincidence that the three most common food allergies are to wheat, corn, and milk. Since supermarkets can now offer a year-round, breath-taking array of foods, the array of literally breath-taking food allergies has grown exponentially.

Grow Out of It—No Way!

Contrary to a lot of common wisdom, children do not grow out of their allergies. In the words of nutritionist Joyce Virtue (who specializes in allergies and food sensitivities), "They simply become allergic adults."

Of course, their symptoms may change. Whereas a child may manifest an allergy by sneezing, coughing, running nose, etc.—that same person may manifest his allergy with depression and other emotional symptoms in adult life.

Pollution further helps provoke allergies. All the junk in our food, air, and water is a constant assault on the body's ability to handle toxins. Our defenses must constantly be on the alert. They go into battle so much, our immune system is compromised. It grows even more defensive—shell-shocked or punch drunk, you might say—and assumes a fighting stance (allergic response) against foods that, under normal circumstances, we'd be able to handle without a problem—or with less of a problem.*

The same over-sensitivity and tendency towards allergy occurs if the first allergy goes unnoticed and is allowed to progress untreated—further compromising and sensitizing the immune system. If your child just has to have his toast every morning, and you give him all he wants—and he keeps on asking for it—chances are good that he is addicted/allergic to it. That allergy may be setting him up for other sensitivities, as well.

---

*Any noxious fumes or pungent, man-made chemicals likely to be used in or around the home may be a culprit in aggravating or potentiating a food allergy or sensitivity. These include: fumes from gas stoves and heaters; waxes; automobile exhaust; disinfectants; cigarette smoke; insecticides; herbicides; aerosol propellants; glue; paint; particle board; paneling; fiberglass insulation; mothballs; nail polish remover; foam rubber; synthetic fabrics in carpets, drapes, and clothes; plastics and other petrochemicals; dust; and pet dander. Joyce Virtue told me that when she fails to find a strong food reaction in a person displaying allergic symptoms, she always investigates the person's environment for allergy-producing factors.

What Are the Symptoms of Food Allergies?

As I said before, if there is any food you or your child "cannot seem to give up," you can justifiably suspect an allergy/addiction to that food.

Babies and young children who drool a lot may have allergies.

If a child is wetting his bed, suspect a food allergy. The offending food is irritating the child's bladder and urethra.

Emotional problems, such as depression and irritability, can be caused by food allergies.

If a child has a tell-tale crease on his nose about three-fourths of the way down, chances are good he has an allergy. The crease is from his constantly wiping his running nose.

Allergic shiners, or dark circles under the eyes, can be a sign of food allergy or sensitivity in children and adults if the person is otherwise eating and sleeping OK.

Hyperactivity is almost always an allergic reaction to chemical additives in food.

Other symptoms of food allergies include: red cheeks, crusty eyes, hay fever, sneezing attacks, frequent sore throats, itching ears and nose, ringing ears, itching eyes, excessively watering eyes, red and swollen eyes, excessive amounts of gas after eating, bloated feeling after meals, heartburn or belching after meals, nausea after meals, chest pains and asthma attacks, joint stiffness and soreness without exercise or exertion, muscle cramps or aches, easily brought on fatigue, itching skin after eating, acne or eczema, and difficulty concentrating. *All are potential symptoms of food allergies or sensitivities.*

Are There Tests To Uncover or Confirm Allergies?

There is a medical lab test to detect food allergies and sensitivities called the cytotoxic blood test. A sample of the blood to be tested is drawn and applied to over 180 different laboratory microscope slides. Then the blood samples on the slides are exposed to concentrated samples of different foods.

The foods that cause toxic reactions—usually white blood cell destruction—in the blood samples, are judged allergenic. The test demonstrates that these foods can act as toxins in your body.

The cytotoxic blood test is currently the best medical test for detecting food sensitivities. The scratch test, which is the favorite of medical allergists, would leave your arm feeling like a pin cushion if you were tested for as many substances as the cytotoxic test covers with only one blood sample. Also, food allergies and sensitivities often do not show up on scratch tests and other tests commonly used by allergists.

Unfortunately, many allergists have not yet embraced the superiority of the cytotoxic test for determining food allergies. This can lead to some unfortunate mistakes. If a child who is hyperactive or who wets the bed or who has emotional symptoms does not show any positive signs of allergies on the scratch or RAST tests, allergists will often refer the child to a psychiatrist. A cytotoxic test might uncover a food allergy or sensitivity that—once treated—could eliminate the problem in a matter of weeks!

The drawback to the cytotoxic test is that it is not (at this writing) available in every city in the country. Compounding this drawback is the fact that the test must be administered before the blood sample is twenty-four hours old.

This factor does not rule out the test for persons living in an area where the test is not available. The same modern transportation system that transports "unseasonal" foods to us all year-round can also transport blood samples from coast-to-coast in a matter of a few hours.

The following is a medical lab that can perform the cytotoxic blood test. It is equipped to refer people to doctors who will help interpret their results and treat them accordingly. This lab is also equipped to handle tests for people thousands of miles away:

Doug Kaufmann, Physicians Labs
1910 Centinela Avenue
Los Angeles, Calif. 90064
Phone: 213-820-4336.

There is another way you can find out if you and your child have food allergies. You can simply rotate your diet. The basic principle of a rotational diet is not to have the same food more than once in any four-day period. (Some rotation diets work on a three, five, six, or seven day period.) During that four-day period, only two or three different foods are eaten at each meal—and those items are not repeated in the diet again for at least four days.

Pay extremely close attention to any symptoms that develop after meals. Make detailed notations. Then, as you proceed, reintroduce foods every four or five days and make note of any changes in symptoms.

The object of the rotation diet is to isolate the food or foods that are causing the symptoms. Once you have your list of "suspect foods," you can test yourself to confirm your suspicions. Reintroduce the suspects one at a time and make note of the symptoms. If you or your child experience a recurrence of symptoms when the suspect foods are introduced, you'll know what's causing your allergic response.

The following is a four-day rotation diet developed by Joyce Virtue for me:*

Day One

Breakfast: Oats and peaches
Lunch: Tuna, lettuce, radishes, cucumbers
Dinner: Halibut, rice, green beans

Day Two

Breakfast: Bananas, cashews
Lunch: Salmon, endive, asparagus, celery
Dinner: Chicken, sweet potatoes, swiss chard

Day Three

Breakfast: Whole wheat cereal, blueberries
Lunch: Turkey, avocado, alfalfa sprouts
Dinner: Lamb, wild rice, zucchini

Day Four

Breakfast: Papaya
Lunch: Sardines, rice cakes, carrots, raw turnips
Dinner: Swordfish, corn on the cob, spinach salad with water chestnuts

---

*Since I had already taken a cytotoxic blood test, Dr. Virtue had some indication of what I was sensitive to when she made up this diet. Thus, some foods appear more than once during the four-day period.

How Do We Treat a Food Allergy?

Once you know what food or foods you and your child are allergic to, you have a choice. Do you totally remove the food or just cut down on it?

Your answer to this question depends on how severe your child's reaction is. If his reaction is very mild, just cutting down on the availability of the food—serving it once a month rather than twice a week—may eliminate the problem. However, if the reaction is severe, you may need to totally eliminate the offending food—not only to treat the present allergy, but also to prevent additional ones from forming while his immune system is compromised.

Rotation of the family diet—or a passionate devotion to *variety*—is not only the key to preventing food allergies, but also to treating them. I heartily recommend variety in your natural foods diet *as a matter of course, whether or not your family has any food allergies or sensitivities.* Many people have told me (as did nutritionists I consulted in preparing this chapter) that they feel so good while on the rotation diet that they permanently incorporate it into their lives!

If Your Child Is Special, He Can Lead the Family

If your child suffers from a severe food allergy, I recommend that the entire family share his special diet. That means if Johnnie has to give up wheat or corn, everybody follows his lead. There are two reasons for this. First, if Johnnie's diet is different from the family's, he'll feel ostracized. That's not good. Second, allergies and food sensitivities tend to run in families. The chances are excellent that following Johnnie's special diet will lead other members of the family—who unwittingly share his allergy—to better health.

As in all other adventures and challenges in this book, your attitude and commitment are vital to the success of your child's special diet. Unless you're positive and totally committed, your child's success will be limited. Every nutritionist I talked to told me sad, sad stories of children whose enthusiasm and successful attempts at changing their diets were ultimately sabotaged by parents who were not totally committed.

Your first goal can be to encourage your allergic child to feel special in a positive way. His specialness is an opportunity for special growth and awareness. The rest of the family should acknowledge it as a privilege to be able to participate in his specialness.

Special Activities

Have your child keep a food diary. Since food allergies are pretty tricky to nail down and eliminate—common allergenic foods, such as wheat, sometimes seem to be everywhere!—a food diary can be a vital tool in detecting and finally eliminating the offending food.

Make it a game. A detective game. Invent a character to help your child detect the "villain" in the food. He can make drawings in his food diary to depict the continuing adventures of his hero.

Extend the detective game further by having your child read the labels on all foods you're considering for purchase. If he spots an item he's allergic or sensitive to, he can tell you not to purchase the food. He'll feel proud that he's able to accept and fulfill this responsibility for his own health.

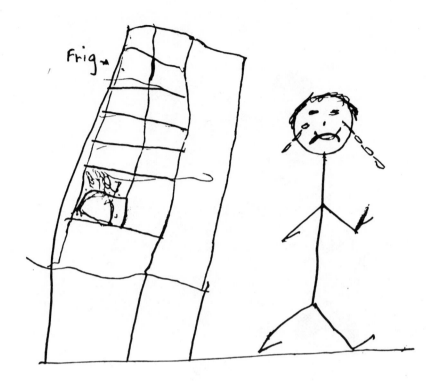

Chocolate Cake

You get chocolate and sprinkle it all around. Put this in the oven and bake it. Put this inside of a refrigerator to get it cold. It tastes nice. I am allergic to chocolate, so I don't eat it anyway.

Dwayne Bugarin

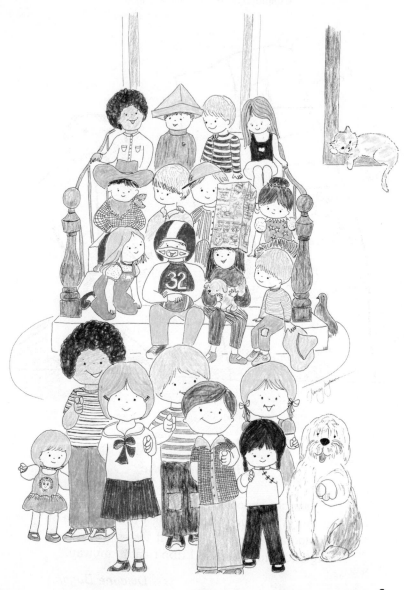

All Children Are Special
--- Including You!

16

For the last 180 pages, I've been sharing with you my ideas on teaching our children. In this chapter, I'd like to share one final thought.

Children are our greatest resource. If we let them, they can teach us so very much. But how about the child still living deep within us adults? That child may be our own greatest personal creative resource. Just as we need to get in touch with our children to teach them, I believe there are great riches in store if we can also get in touch with the child inside each of us. My final thought for this book is: Love the child in yourself.

There's a certain fundamental honesty about natural foods. Take a sprout, for example. A sprout, as you know, is the most intense concentration of creative life force in the plant world. Ounce for ounce, a sprout is alive with more creative juices than any other plant tissue.

Children are like sprouts. They're so alive with creativity and vitality that it just bubbles over all the time. And just as a sprout is so beautifully clear and forthright about its purpose, children are gloriously honest about what they see, feel, want, and need.

I'll never forget walking into my classroom one day when a little girl came up to me and said, "Mrs. Gooch, you don't have your clown suit on today!"

I immediately understood that the child was referring to the brightly colored gaily designed, expensive dress I'd worn the previous day. The little girl wasn't teasing me. In her eyes, my outfit was a clown suit—and that was just fine with her. Her observation was expressed without the slightest hesitation. Not only did she accept my "clown suit," but she wanted me to wear it again!

Children are so direct. You don't have to try to figure them out. They're right up front. They'll just come sit next to you and say, "I love you!" or "That's an ugly dress!" or "Your breath smells!" or "Please hug me! I need a hug!"

Children are also really in tune with their appetites and sensations. They know when they're full, and they push the plate away. They know when they're hungry, and they find something to eat. They know when they're happy and when they're sad—and they let us know about it in no uncertain terms! All too often, however, we don't hear them.

On the broad scale of what we want and need out of life, children are more up front with themselves, as well as with us. When a child wants something, it's a very simple matter: "I want that!" The child doesn't have to think up eighteen reasons why she wants it. She just wants it. And that's enough for her.

It's we parents who teach our children to stifle these qualities. After all, we have learned that "it doesn't always pay to be so honest" and "you really do have to put off satisfying your deepest needs and desires" and "you do need eighteen reasons to justify wanting something."

I know, it's one thing to be up front with yourself and openly admit all your needs and desires—and another to acknowledge that we can't always have things the way we want them at exactly the moment when we want them!

And that is precisely my point. They are two entirely different things. I'm afraid that what happens is we teach ourselves and our children that just because we can't always satisfy our wants, that we also shouldn't be honest about them. And I don't believe that's true at all.

When we tune out our wants and needs, we lose that vital, life-giving quality that children display. We forget how to be up front with ourselves, because "it's not always best." We "grow up." We lose touch with the child inside of us. That's bad enough, but then we encourage our children to do the same thing.

I have written this book to help us get in closer touch with our children, so that we might teach them some of the important things we want them to learn. In Chapter 3, I said that "teaching is an act of love." Whether we consciously think of it that way or not, the act of teaching cannot be dissociated from acceptance, responsibility, affirmation, honesty, freedom, and fun.

Those six principles will help us achieve that openness for communication and receptivity that we need if we are to help, support, and teach anyone. I also believe that these six principles can help us love our children, too.

But now, we need to add one more principle, one more act of love that will increase our effectiveness in teaching our children. We need to *love the child in ourselves.*

We need to apply these six principles to ourselves to get in tune with the beautiful child-like qualities of honesty, vitality, creativity, and love that are inside us all—but which we have allowed to be buried under the accumulated "wisdom" of adulthood.

I believe that if we try our best to achieve the honesty, simplicity, and enthusiasm of a child's approach to life, we will not only be more effective teachers of our children, but we will also accomplish more in our own lives and loves.

One Final Special Activity:
Turn the Tables—Love the Child in You!

We parents should switch roles with our children now and then. This activity is a reverse-image mirror on all of the special activities in this book. Let your child be the teacher/parent sometimes. Let her know that she is so special that you trust her as much as she has to trust you.

This activity is also great for getting an honest, child's-eye view of what you look like as you go about your job as parent/teacher. Your child becomes a living mirror of you. Notice what steps she emphasizes. Notice her gestures and attitude, her tone of voice and style. She is portraying the way *you* appear to her.

And you become a living mirror of her. Please be mindful of how important your view of her is to your child's developing self-esteem. She really needs you to like what you see in her.

Get in touch with the child in you. Take a walk alone. Think about all the things you've wanted and felt in your life, all your deepest desires and fears. Allow yourself to share any and all information in you *with yourself.* Allow yourself to admit that you do want a lot and that there is a lot of pure feeling inside of you. That is the child in you. That is the you that may have been hidden by growing up, but who has always been with you.

Your own son or daughter has that well of deep feeling, too—only our children are much closer to it than we are. If you can experience that well of deep, pure feeling in yourself, it will be that much easier for you to understand and mirror your child's feelings.

I believe that when we love the child in ourselves, we can better love our own children. We can, after all, say to ourselves, too: "If you love me, don't feed *me* junk!"

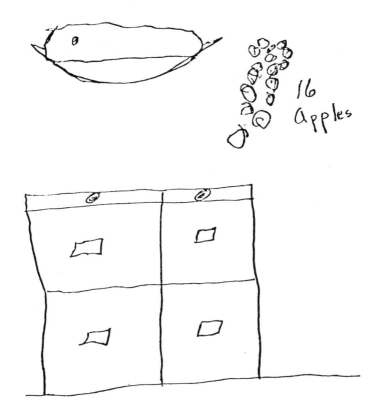

Apple Pie

To make dough, you need 3 or 2 cups of butter, 1 cup of water and 3 cups of flour. Pat the dough down, and put it in a pan. Cut it if it is too long.

The filling consists of: a whole bunch of butter, about 6 spoons of honey, and 9 or 10 or 16 apples. (The red has to be out of them.) Cook this on the stove for 15 minutes, unless you have 16 apples. Then you would cook it for 16 minutes. Put on some pink cake frosting and pop it in the oven at 40°. Serve this with Cool Whip, or if you really feel spunky you can whip up some cream.

Mike Bjornson

Appendix A

The Elements of Whole Food

Protein

Protein is the building block of the body, the raw material for all growth, repair, and maintenance. Every organ and body fluid requires protein. So, when there's not enough protein in the diet, the whole body suffers.

Although there are over one thousand different proteins in the body, they are made up of different combinations of simpler molecules called amino acids. The body can make twelve of the twenty amino acids by itself. The remaining eight must be supplied through the food we eat. Excess protein is stored as fat or burned for energy.

Carbohydrates

Carbohydrates are the starches and sugars that supply us with energy. The body breaks down all starches and sugars into glucose, or blood sugar. Glucose serves as fuel for the cells that make up the tissues of the body and that carry out its many functions.

Carbohydrates are best used by the body when they are accompanied by specific nutrients that aid in their digestion. The "carbohydrate team" consists of not only carbohydrates, but also B vitamins, certain minerals, and enzymes. Sometimes these accessory members of the team are missing, as in the case of refined carbohydrates like white sugar and white flour. When these vitamins, minerals, and enzymes aren't present, the body "borrows" them from other teams, which puts undue stress on the other teams. If the supply from the other teams runs out, our body's supply of energy runs low. Eventually, other body systems that rely on B vitamins and minerals also suffer.

The total carbohydrate team is present in whole foods such as whole wheat, brown rice, and other whole grains. In the refined carbohydrates, the accessory factors are mostly absent.

Fats

Fat serves as the body's reserve energy supply, as a co-factor in many metabolic reactions, and as a structural element in the cells. As with carbohydrates and protein, excess fat in the diet is stored in the body. Stored fat is converted to energy when the need arises. Naturally, we do not want too many excess fat players stored on our "playing field," since they can eventually make the game more difficult and less fun for all the others players—including us!

Vitamins and Minerals

There are almost three dozen team members that come under the heading of vitamins and minerals. These are called "micronutrients" because they are supplied in much smaller quantities than the "macronutrients" such as protein and carbohydrates. A child may eat twenty to forty grams of protein a day, for example, but hardly more than a gram or two of all the micronutrients combined.

Nevertheless, the micronutrients are every bit as important as the macronutrients. The micronutrients act as accessory factors, supplying crucial biochemicals at key points in metabolic chain reactions. The absence of one or more micronutrients will eventually lead to poor performance on the part of the entire team. All of the micronutrients must be brought into the game from outside, through the diet. The body cannot manufacture them.

The following is only a brief discussion of the basic role of each vitamin and mineral in the health of our body. For a more elaborate explanation, I have recommended several books in Appendix C.

[*Note:* When buying chewable vitamins, beware of formulas that contain sugar, sucrose, fructose, starch, or artificial colors. Chewable vitamins sweetened with orange juice are available.]

Vitamins

Vitamin A

Vitamin A promotes the health of our eyes, skin, bones, teeth, mucous membranes, adrenal glands (which govern our response to stress), and the glands which secrete digestive juices. We need vitamin A to resist infection, grow, heal wounds, and adjust our eyesight to darkness. Food sources of vitamin A include yellow and orange vegetables, tomatoes, dark green leafy vegetables, liver, egg yolk, and dairy products.

Thiamine (B1)

Thiamine's main job on the Health Team is to make possible the production of energy from the digestion of carbohydrates. Since the brain's demand for energy is so high, mental alertness and emotional health require a diet with enough thiamine. Organ meats (liver, kidney, heart), yeast, lean meat, eggs, green leafy vegetables, whole grains, nuts, berries, and legumes are the best food sources of thiamine.

Riboflavin (B2)

Riboflavin is central to the body's utilization of protein, fats, carbohydrates, and the other B vitamins. All of the cells of the body require riboflavin in order to transfer nutrients across the cell membrane. The health of the eyes, skin, and nails depend on riboflavin. Food sources include organ meats, fish, dairy products, eggs, green leafy vegetables, wheat germ, whole grains, and legumes.

Niacin (B3)

A cell's ability to utilize all major nutrients depends on niacin. The brain, nervous system, skin, and digestive system are particularly dependent on an adequate supply of niacin. Food sources include organ meats, fish, yeast, whole grains, dried peas and beans, and nuts.

Pyridoxine (B6)

This team member is central to the body's use of protein, fat, and carbohydrates. Energy production, all growing tissue, the liver and the heart, and the entire nervous system depend on an adequate supply of this vitamin. Food sources include liver and other organ meats, whole grains, wheat germ, soybeans, yeast, corn, blackstrap molasses, cabbage, bananas, potatoes, avocados, peas, and green peppers.

Folic Acid

All the cells of the body require folic acid in order to grow and reproduce. Folic acid teams up with vitamins C and B12 to use protein and maintain a healthy nervous system. The red blood cells, bone marrow, hair, fingernails, immune system, mucous membranes, liver, and nervous system depend on an adequate supply of folic acid. Food sources include organ meats, dark green leafy vegetables, asparagus, yeast, whole grains, wheat germ, lentils, lima beans, and orange juice.

B12 (Cobalamin)

This team member is necessary for cell reproduction. The red blood cells and the nervous system will not function properly without adequate B12. Folic acid cannot be utilized by the body unless B12 is supplied in adequate quantities. Food sources include organ meats, yeast, wheat germ, sea vegetables (wakame, kombu), and soybeans.

Pantothenic Acid

Our response to stress depends on this team member, which supports the adrenal glands and nervous system. Sources of pantothenic acid include organ meats, egg yolk, peanuts, broccoli, cauliflower, cabbage, whole grains, and bran.

Biotin

The body's use of protein, fat, carbohydrates, folic acid, and pantothenic acid depends on biotin. The skin, thyroid gland, adrenals, reproductive tract, and nervous system are particularly dependent on this member of the Health Team. Sources include organ meats, egg yolk, peanuts, filberts, mushrooms, cauliflower, and whole grains.

Choline

The transmission of nervous impulses depends on a chemical that is derived from choline. Thus, the function of the nervous system and also the liver depend on the presence of this team member. Sources include lecithin, whole grains, yeast, fish, eggs, legumes, and liver.

Inositol

Inositol is vital to the health of brain cells, bone marrow, the eyes, and the intestines. Also, without adequate inositol, the body cannot metabolize dietary fat. Food sources include lecithin, yeast, liver, whole grains, nuts, fruit, and vegetables.

PABA (Para-Amino-Benzoic Acid)

PABA aids in the synthesis of two other team members, folic acid and pantothenic acid. The health of the skin, hair, and digestive tract depend on this vitamin. Sources include yeast, liver, and whole grains.

Vitamin C

Vitamin C is one of the superstars of the Health Team. It seems to have an important role in several vital "plays," including: the formation of collagen and other fibrous tissue (skin, tendons, bone, teeth, cartilage, and connective tissue), the metabolism of protein, wound healing, the strength of blood vessels, the strength of the immune system, and the strength of the adrenal glands. Food sources include citrus fruits, strawberries, cantaloupes, and raw vegetables (especially peppers, parsley, broccoli, cauliflower, kale, brussels sprouts, turnip greens, cabbage, tomatoes, potatoes, and bean sprouts).

Vitamin D

Vitamin D makes possible the absorption and proper utilization of calcium and phosphorus—minerals which are required for strong bones and teeth. Natural sources include sunshine (the body manufactures vitamin D upon exposure to adequate sunshine), fish, liver, egg yolk, and summer milk.

Vitamin E

This team member protects the membranes of all the cells from oxidizing and dying prematurely. The skin, reproductive system, muscles, and red blood cells are particularly dependent on vitamin E. Sources include whole grains, seeds, nuts, eggs, fish, and organ meats.

Minerals

Calcium

Calcium is the mineral that makes the bones and teeth hard and strong. This team member is also required for the normal function of muscles and nerves. Sources include milk, egg yolk, fish (small fish, eaten with the bones—like sardines), soybeans, green leafy vegetables, roots, tubers, and seeds.

Chromium

Chromium works in tandem with the hormone insulin to use blood sugar to produce energy. Protein and fat metabolism also depend upon this mineral, as does cell reproduction. Sources include brewer's yeast, whole grains, blackstrap molasses, black pepper, liver, cheese, sea food, meat, and nuts.

Copper

Copper is required for the production of energy in the cells; the utilization of iron; the strength of the myelin sheath that protects the nerves; and the formation of collagen, melanin (pigment), and elastin (the substance that lends elasticity to the tissues). Sources include bran, mushrooms, peas, leafy vegetables, legumes, nuts, seafood, poultry, and whole grains.

Iodine

The formation of the thyroid hormone, which regulates the body's metabolic rate, depends on iodine. Sources include seafood and seaweed.

Iron

The chief role of this team member is to produce hemoglobin, the red substance that enables the blood cells to carry oxygen to the body's cells and carbon dioxide away from them. Sources include liver, heart, kidney, lean meat, shellfish, dried beans and fruits, nuts, green leafy vegetables, whole grains, and blackstrap molasses.

Magnesium

This mineral plays a pivotal role in regulating all the vital functions of the cells, including metabolism and reproduction. It is also required for the health of the muscles and nervous system. Sources include legumes, nuts, whole grains, and shellfish.

Manganese

Manganese is required for protein synthesis, formation of cartilage, cell reproduction, fat metabolism, and the utilization of insulin to produce energy. Sources include whole grains, wheat germ, bran, peas, tea, ginger, sage, nuts, and leafy vegetables.

Molybdenum

This mineral is required, in trace amounts, for the production of energy. Sources include legumes, organ meats, milk, and grains.

Phosphorus

Every metabolic process in the body requires phosphorus, including energy production, carbohydrate-fat-protein utilization, blood chemistry, and nervous tissue function. The strength of the bones and teeth also depends on phosphorus. Sources include meat, fish, poultry, eggs, milk, cheese, nuts, and legumes.

Potassium

Nerve excitation, muscular contraction, and cellular metabolism require potassium. Adequate supplies of potassium are also required for regular heartbeat, muscle coordination, and strength. Sources include bananas, lettuce, broccoli, potatoes, fresh fruit, peanuts, wheat germ, squash, nuts, and orange juice.

Selenium

This team member is necessary for the health of the muscles and blood, and the detoxification of poisonous metals (such as mercury) that pollute our environment. Selenium is also required for cellular functions; reproductive functions; and the strength of the skin, hair, nails, and immune system. Sources include organ meats, whole grains, and brewer's yeast.

Silicon

Silicon is required for the maintenance of connective tissue and bone, for healing, and for embryonic development. Sources include whole grains, fruits, and vegetables.

Sodium

Sodium is the team member that makes it possible to "pump" fluids in and out of the cells. Sodium chloride, or regular table salt, is the best source.

Zinc

Zinc is another superstar of the Health Team. It is a crucial factor in every body function that depends on enzymes. These body functions include reproduction and growth, protein synthesis, formation of connective tissue, protection of cell membranes, metabolism of other minerals, and the health of the immune system and reproductive system. Sources include seafood, liver, meat, milk, eggs, nuts, legumes, and brewer's yeast.

Other Factors

With older children, you can further emphasize the importance of a diet of whole, natural foods by pointing out that there are several team players whose existence are suspected—but whose identities are not yet known. Nutritionists call these players "X Factors." One example of evidence of the existence of these factors is sea water. Scientists can chemically duplicate sea water, but their artificial variety will not sustain aquatic life. This suggests that there are unknown factors present in the Real Thing. Therefore, you can logically reason that a diet of manufactured food may supply most of the known players—but will be deficient in the X Factors.

You can also use the team concept to teach your child some additional concepts in nutrition, such as the need for fiber. Fiber, available in whole grains, fruits, and vegetables, provides mechanical bulk that keeps our digestion and elimination working properly in much the same way that an offensive lineman provides the bulk that enables the quarterback to keep moving.

Food storage, cooking, and processing can be explained to your child in terms of adding unwanted team players (through processing) or taking away necessary ones (through cooking, storage, and processing). Thus, you can use the team concept to demonstrate the effects of each of these factors on food and health.

Appendix B

Natural Foods Recipes
and
Substitution Guide

Cooking Hints

Sweeteners

Three-quarters cup **honey** can be used in place of one cup sugar. As a rule, reduce the liquid in the recipe by one-half cup for every cup of honey, and bake at a temperature 25 degrees lower than the original instructions indicate.

Three-quarters cup of **maple syrup** can be substituted for one cup sugar. Reduce the liquid by two tablespoons.

Date sugar can be substituted in equal parts for sugar. To keep date sugar soft, store in a covered container with a piece of bread. Refined fructose, high-fructose corn syrup, and turbinado sugar are not natural foods.

Salt

There are several salt substitutes on the market, most of which do, however, contain some salt (sodium chloride) or potassium salt (potassium chloride). Parsley Patch Pure Spice Company (P.O. Box 2043, Santa Rosa, Calif. 95405) markets seven totally salt-free natural spice blends which I recommend not only to people who wish to cut down or totally eliminate salt from their diets but also to everyone who wants to season their food with gourmet quality natural spices. Parsely Patch uses a total of twenty-nine herbs and spices in seven combinations—French, Italian, Mexican, Oriental, Winter Spice, Curry, and All Purpose.

Shortenings and Margarine

You can use straight butter as a substitute for shortening, but to approximate the consistency of the shortening in a recipe, you can use butter mixed with oil. Use one-third cup oil and one-half cup butter for each one cup shortening called for in the original recipe.

Gelatin Dessert

For each tablespoon of artificially flavored gelatin dessert, use one tablespoon of plain gelatin or agar-agar and a pint of unsweetened fruit juice. Use fruit juice instead of water and heat as you would the water. Add fresh fruit, if desired.

Coffee

You can use a soy or barley grain brew coffee substitute (such as Duram Un-coffee or Sipp) to substitute for coffee.

Chocolate

If your favorite chocolate cake calls for cocoa, simply use an equal amount of carob powder. If it calls for baking chocolate, use three tablespoons of carob powder plus one tablespoon each of water and vegetable oil as a substitute for one square of chocolate. Since carob is high in natural sugars, use less sweetener when you substitute it for cocoa.

Flour

Whole wheat pastry flour (a finer grind than regular whole wheat flour) can be substituted on a one-to-one basis for cake flour or all-purpose flour. Other whole grain flours, such as rye, triticale, rice, or soy, may also be substituted on an equal basis. You may want to sift the whole grain flours three or four times to lighten them, however.

Cornstarch

Natural alternatives to corn starch include arrowroot powder, tapioca, whole wheat flour, and brown rice flour, substituted on a one-to-one basis.

Baking Powder

Low-sodium baking powder can be substituted in equal amounts for regular baking powder. **Active dry yeast** can also be used, but you must use warm liquids in the recipe to activate the yeast. **Cream of tartar** can also be substituted for baking powder in a ratio of one-half tartar to one baking powder.

If you want to use **baking soda** in recipes instead of baking powder, you must add an acid food to react with the soda and produce carbon dioxide gas to leaven your recipe. For one teaspoon baking powder in a recipe, substitute one-half teaspoon baking soda plus one and one-half teaspoons lemon juice or vinegar. If your recipe calls for milk, you can use one-half teaspoon baking soda and one-half cup buttermilk (in place of one-half cup of the regular milk) as a substitute for baking powder.

Oats

Rolled oats are sometimes too coarse to be used in oatmeal cookies. Chop them briefly in a blender before using.

Liquids

One cup milk equals four tablespoons dry milk powder plus one cup water, soy milk, or fruit juice. You can use fruit juice, soup stock, milk, or yogurt as a substitute for water, too.

Buttermilk

To make buttermilk, or sour milk, add two tablespoons lemon juice to one cup sweet milk. Let stand for five minutes.

Herbs

One-quarter teaspoon dried herbs equals one teaspoon minced fresh herbs. If cooking time is more than one hour, add herbs for just the last hour.

Beans

One cup dried beans equals two and one-half cups cooked beans. *Tip:* Savory, an herb, eliminates the gas produced by beans.

How To Convert a Recipe

Basic Oatmeal Cookies

Original Recipe	Converted Recipe
1 cup shortening	1/2 cup butter plus 1/3 cup oil
1 cup brown sugar	1/2 cup molasses
1 cup white sugar	1/2 cup honey
2 eggs, beaten	2 eggs, beaten
1 teaspoon vanilla	1 teaspoon vanilla
1 1/2 cups all-purpose flour	1 1/2 cups whole wheat pastry flour
1 teaspoon salt	1 teaspoon salt
1 teaspoon baking soda	1 teaspoon baking soda (or omit)
3 cups rolled oats	3 cups rolled oats (ground in blender)

Cream shortening and sugars together. Beat in eggs and vanilla. Combine flour, salt, and soda, mixing well. Add flour mixture and oats to wet mixture. Drop by teaspoonfuls onto lightly oiled cookie sheet, leaving about two inches between cookies. Flatten with a wet fork. Bake in preheated 350 degree oven for 10 minutes. Cool on rack.

Chop butter into flour. Add oil, mixing it in lightly with a fork. Add oats and salt. Work the mixture lightly with your fingers as you would pastry. In a small bowl, combine eggs, molasses, honey, and vanilla. Stir this wet mixture into the dry ingredients and mix. Drop by teaspoonfuls onto lightly oiled cookie sheet, leaving two inches between cookies. Flatten with a wet fork. Bake in preheated 325 degree oven for 10 minutes. Cool on rack.

Carob Raisin Cookies

This is a simple recipe that I like to bake for Harry's two daughters.

1/2 cup softened butter
1 cup light honey
2 eggs, slightly beaten
2 1/2 cups whole wheat pastry flour, sifted twice
1 teaspoon vanilla
1 teaspoon baking soda
1 cup chopped nuts (optional)
1 cup carob-coated raisins
    (or carob chips and raisins)

Cream butter and honey. Add eggs and other ingredients. Mix heartily, then chill the dough for at least three hours. Drop by teaspoonfuls onto an oiled cookie sheet. Bake at 350 degrees for about 10 minutes.

Oat Crisps

2/3 cup butter
1/2 cup honey
2 cups old fashioned oats
1 cup grated coconut
1/2 teaspoon cinnamon
1 teaspoon vanilla
1 teaspoon grated lemon rind
1 teaspoon grated orange rind
1/2 teaspoon salt
1/4 cup whole wheat pastry flour

Cream butter with honey. Add all remaining ingredients. Mix well. Form into 2 rectangles approximately 1″ by 2″. Chill in freezer until completely firm. Cut into 1/4-inch sticks. Bake at 300 degrees about 20 minutes, or until cookies are lightly browned. Cool before removing from cookie sheets.

Walnut Short Bread Cookies

1/2 cup butter
1/4 cup honey
2 teaspoons vanilla
1 1/4 cups whole wheat pastry flour
1 tablespoon dry milk powder
1 cup walnuts (finely chopped)

Cream together butter and honey. Add vanilla. Stir in sifted flour with dry milk powder. Add walnuts. (Dough should be somewhat stiff.) Divide dough in half and roll each half on waxed paper to make long, narrow roll. Flatten sides to form long rectangle. Wrap waxed paper around log and place in freezer. When ready to bake, preheat oven to 275 degrees. Slice cookies about 1/2 inch thick. Bake approximately 40 minutes. *Watch out for too much browning on the bottom if oven is too hot!*

Carob Cream Dream Candy

3-ounces cream cheese
1/2 cup honey
2 teaspoons carob powder
3/4 cup toasted wheat germ
1 teaspoon vanilla
1/3 cup chopped walnuts and pecans, combined
ground coconut and pecans (for rolling candy)

Combine ingredients, mixing well with fork. Shape into balls and roll in coconut and pecan meal. Some may be rolled separately in either coconut meal or pecan meal.

Auntie Sue's Whole Wheat Bread

All ingredients should be at room temperature, unless otherwise stated. Let your child feel and smell all the ingredients as they're added.

Combine in a large bowl:

3 cups warm water
3/4 cup honey
3 tablespoons dry baker's yeast, or three yeast cakes.

Allow yeast to soften in mixture for five minutes or so, then add:

1/4 cup safflower oil
4 cups unsifted stone ground whole wheat flour
1 cup soy flour
1 scant teaspoon salt

1. Beat by hand 100 or more strokes. If the dough is not beaten sufficiently, the bread will be too heavy.
2. Add and stir well 2 to 3 cups whole wheat flour, enough to make the dough stiff.
3. Sprinkle approximately 1 cup whole wheat flour on board and turn dough out on it.
4. Knead until dough is smooth and elastic (7 to 10 minutes). Use more flour if required to prevent sticking.
5. Put dough into oiled bowl, smooth side down. Then, turn greased side up.
6. Cover and let rise in a warm place until it doubles in size.
7. When doubled, knead or push down to original size. Cover and let rise again for about 60-90 minutes, or until double in bulk.
8. Knead one more time.
9. Divide kneaded dough into three parts, and shape loaves into three greased loaf pans.
10. Bake in 350 degree oven about 50 minutes. (If divided into two loaves, bake about 70 minutes.)
11. Turn out on wire racks to cool.

Option: Loaves can be brushed with beaten egg whites and sprinkled with sesame or poppy seeds before baking.

Matthew Levanthal's Pumpkin Bread

Nine year old Matt was one of my most cherished students. He converted this recipe and baked it all by himself—and won First Prize in the bread division of Mrs. Gooch's First Bake Off! I was so proud of him, and he had a grin from ear to ear, too! (A panel of professional judges chose his recipe over all the others. My vote didn't count.)

3 1/2 cups sifted whole wheat flour
2 teaspoons baking soda
1 1/2 teaspoons salt
1 teaspoon cinnamon
1 teaspoon nutmeg

Put in a large bowl and make a hole in the middle of it. Add the following in the middle and mix well:

1 1/2 cups honey
1 cup oil
4 eggs
3/4 cup water
1 16-ounce can pumpkin filling
1 cup chopped walnuts

Pour into two greased and floured loaf pans. Bake at 350 degrees for 1 hour and 15 minutes. Serve hot or cold, plain, or with butter or honey butter.

Apple Tart

Crust:

1 1/4 cups whole wheat pastry flour
1/3 cup wheat germ
1/2 teaspoon salt
1/2 cup butter
1 egg yolk
1 teaspoon grated lemon rind
1 tablespoon lemon juice
2 tablespoons honey

Filling:

6 cups sliced, pared tart apples
1/4 cup whole wheat pastry flour
1/4 cup honey
1/2 teaspoon cinnamon
1 teaspoon vanilla
3/4 cup natural apricot preserves

Mix flour, wheat germ, and salt. Cut in butter until mixture is crumbly. Mix egg yolk with honey, lemon peel and juice. Add to flour mixture, and blend. Pat into bottom and two inches up side of nine-inch spring-form pan. Mix apples with flour, honey, cinnamon, and vanilla. Turn into pastry-lined pan. Arrange some apple slices decoratively on top, if desired. Spread apricot preserves over apples. Bake tart about 1 hour at 350 degrees, or until apples are tender. Serve with whipped cream.

Quiche Lorraine

2 cups milk or half-and-half
2 cups shredded swiss cheese
3/4 cup onion
4 eggs
1 teaspoon salt
dash cayenne pepper
dash nutmeg
1 teaspoon honey

Crust:

1 1/2 cup whole wheat flour
1 cup raw butter
4 tablespoons cold water
1 teaspoon salt

Mix crust ingredients together, and press into pie plate. Mix remaining ingredients, and pour into crust. Bake at 425 degrees for 1/2 hour.

Cranberry Orange Torte

This recipe was converted by Matthew Levanthal's mother, Nancy. It won First Prize in the cake division of Mrs. Gooch's First Bake Off.

Sift together:

2 1/4 cups sifted whole wheat flour
1 1/2 teaspoons baking soda
1/2 teaspoon salt

Add to the above mixture and stir:

grated rind of two oranges
1 cup chopped dates (use scissors)
1 cup chopped walnuts
1 cup cranberries (fresh)

Mix and add to the above mixture:

2 eggs, beaten
1 cup buttermilk
3/4 cup oil
1/2 cup honey

Preheat oven to 350 degrees. Grease and flour pan. Add mixture, and bake 50 minutes to 1 hour. (Makes 2 small loaf pans or one bundt cake.) Remove from oven when done. Let cool until lukewarm. Remove from pan, but return to pan when cool to add "topping."

"Topping:" Mix one cup orange juice with 1/2 cup honey. Pour mixture over cooled cake while still in pan. Cake will soak up just about all of it. Remove and wrap in foil. Refrigerate. Serve with whipped cream: (1/2 pint whipping cream, 1 teaspoon vanilla, 1 tablespoon honey) and orange garnish. Will keep 7 to 10 days. Can be remoistened with orange juice before serving.

Date Cake

1 cup pitted dates, cut into sixths
1 cup water
1/2 teaspoon soda
1/2 cup butter
1/2 cup honey
2 eggs
1 1/2 cups whole wheat pastry flour
1/4 teaspoon cinnamon
1/2 teaspoon baking soda
1 teaspoon vanilla

Place dates in bowl. Bring water to boil and add soda. Stir until soda dissolves. Pour liquid over dates. Cool. Cream together butter and honey. Add eggs to creamed mixture, one at a time. Beat well. Sift flour with baking soda, cinnamon, and salt. Add to creamed mixture alternately with the water poured off the dates. Beat well after each addition. Stir in dates and vanilla. Spread in a well-greased 9-inch square pan. Bake at 325 degrees for 40–50 minutes. When cake is cool, cover with the following topping.

Topping: Boil 3/4 cup honey for about 5 minutes. Add 1/2 cup finely chopped dates, 1/2 cup butter, and 1/2 cup chopped walnuts. Continue cooking until thick. Cool, and pour over cooled cake.

Poppy Seed Cake

1 1/2 cups honey
3/4 cup butter
1 teaspoon vanilla
4 eggs
3 cups whole wheat pastry flour
1/3 cup poppy seeds
2 1/2 teaspoons baking soda
1/2 teaspoon salt
1/2 cup buttermilk
1 medium banana, mashed down to 1/3 cup
1/2 cup raisins
1/4 cup honey

Cream Cheese Topper

1 3-ounce package cream cheese, softened
2 tablespoons butter
1 teaspoon vanilla
1 cup nonfat dry milk powder
toasted sliced almonds

Thoroughly beat together honey, butter, and vanilla until fluffy. Add eggs. Mix flour, poppy seeds, baking soda, and salt. Combine buttermilk and mashed banana. Combine wet and dry ingredients. Stir in raisins. Turn into greased 10-inch fluted tube pan. Bake in 350 degree oven for 50–55 minutes. Cool cake completely.

For Topper: combine wet ingredients and beat until fluffy. Add dry milk powder and beat well. Serve with cake in separate bowl or spread on top.

Pineapple Bran Muffins

1/4 cup drained, unsweetened crushed pineapple, sweetened with
    honey to taste
1 large egg
1 cup milk
3 tablespoons olive or safflower oil
3 tablespoons molasses
3 tablespoons honey
1 teaspoon baking soda
1 teaspoon vinegar
1 heaping cup freshly ground and sifted whole wheat pastry flour
1 heaping cup bran

Mix pineapple and honey. Let stand. In large bowl, beat egg. Add milk, mixing well. Stir in oil, molasses, and honey. In separate bowl, mix baking soda and vinegar, and add to milk mixture. Stir in whole wheat flour. Fold in bran. Spoon mixture into 12 oiled muffin cups. Add 1 teaspoon of pineapple to center of each. Bake at 425 degrees for 12 minutes.

Harry's Pecan Pie

Harry, the Original Junk Food Junkie, converted this recipe himself. He obtained the original recipe from a restaurant in New Orleans. He had a really super time in the kitchen experimenting with the natural substitutions. For my birthday, he had fifty people over for a surprise dinner party—of all natural food. For dessert, we had Harry's Pecan Pie. He had baked eight of them!

Crust:

2 cups sifted whole wheat pastry flour
1/2 cup cold butter
1 1/2 tablespoons oil
1/2 teaspoon salt
5-6 tablespoons ice water

Sift flour and salt. Cut in butter with two knives or pastry cutter. Gradually stir the oil and water into flour mixture. Quickly form into a ball. If it doesn't shape up, add more ice water. Roll out on floured surface. Place in pie pan and fill.

Filling:

5 eggs
1/4 cup melted butter
1 1/4 cup ironbark honey
1 1/4 cup white clover honey
1-2 teaspoons vanilla
1 cup chopped pecans per pie (recipe makes 2 regular 9-inch pies or 3 8-inch pies.

Beat eggs with wire whisk or fork. Add butter, vanilla, and honey. Mix well. Pour mixture into pie shells, filling each about 2/3 full. Sprinkle one cup chopped pecans per pie. Bake at 350 degrees for 50 to 55 minutes—20 minutes with door closed, then 15 minutes with door open (this allows pie to settle), then balance of time with door closed.

Carob Pie

Crust:

1 cup whole wheat pastry flour
1/4 teaspoon salt
1/4 cup sesame oil
1/4 cup water

Filling:

1/2 cup honey
1/2 cup butter
3 tablespoons agar-agar
1/2 cup water
3 tablespoons carob
2 eggs
1 teaspoon vanilla

Mix carob with 2 tablespoons water. Cream together butter and honey. Stir vanilla and carob into the butter-honey mixture. Dissolve agar-agar in 1/2 cup water over low heat, and then let cool slightly. Beat the agar-agar into carob mixture until well-blended. Beat one egg into the mixture; then add the other egg and beat until the color of the mixture changes from dark brown to light brown. If mixture starts to separate, stop beating immediately. (The color won't affect the taste.) Pour mixture into baked pie crust and freeze until firm. Before serving, top with whipped cream.

French's Cheese Cake

Crust:

1 cup whole wheat flour
1/4 cup honey
1/2 teaspoon vanilla
1 egg yolk
1/4 cup butter

Filling:

2 8-ounce packages cream cheese, softened
3 eggs
1 cup honey
2 tsp vanilla
1/2 teaspoon almond extract
3 cups sour cream
pinch of salt

Topping:

3 cups red tart cherries
2 tablespoons honey
2/3 cup corn starch

Crust: Combine ingredients for crust in bowl and beat with fork until smooth. Spread crust directly onto a springform pan, as evenly as possible, with a knife. (Take the pan apart to spread the crust evenly, and put only the bottom of the pan in to bake.) Bake at 400 degrees for 6 to 8 minutes. Put pan back together and put in filling.

Filling: Combine all ingredients for filling in a bowl and beat with an electric beater for about 5 minutes. Pour into baked crust and bake at 250 degrees for about one hour.

Topping: Drain cherry juice into a sauce pan. Add honey and corn-starch and bring mixture to a boil. Let cool slightly, then add the cherries. Let cool. Place on top of cheese cake after it has cooled. Cool completed cheese cake in refrigerator for about 8 hours before serving.

Ten Dollar Cheese Cake

3 pounds cream cheese (6 8-ounce packages)
1 1/4 cups raw honey
4 eggs
1 tablespoon grated lemon peel
pinch sea salt
1 teaspoon vanilla
1/3 cup whipping cream

Crust:

1 1/4 cups whole wheat pastry flour
1/2 cup butter
2 tablespoons milk

Prepare crust by cutting butter into flour until mixture resembles coarse crumbs. Work in milk until dough is soft and forms a ball. Chill. Roll out to fit a 10-inch springform pan. Fit in bottom of pan and trim edges.

Blend cheese and honey until smooth. Add eggs one at a time, blending well after each addition. Add lemon peel and blend. Add salt and vanilla. Blend well. Add cream and blend. Pour into crust-lined pan and top with fruit, if desired. Bake at 325 degrees for 1 1/2 hours. Let cool in oven 1 hour before removing. Cool in refrigerator. Best when aged in refrigerator 24 hours before serving.

Auntie Sue's Crunchy Granola

This is the granola Sue Epstein made with her granddaughters in Germany.

Preheat oven to 350 degrees. In a large bowl or cooking pot, mix:

1/2 cup vegetable oil
2/3 cup honey
1 tablespoon vanilla

Blend this well, then stir in:

8 cups rolled oats
1 1/4 cups sesame seeds
1 cup raw sunflower seeds
2 cups coconut shreds
1/4 cup non-instant milk powder.

Spread mixture in several large, shallow baking pans. Be sure to spread evenly. Bake 20-25 minutes, or until lightly browned. Check and stir often. Makes 12 cups. One cup yields about 9 grams of protein.

Options: Add chopped or sliced almonds or walnuts, cinnamon, dried chopped apples, or raisins.

School Lunch Ideas

Sandwich Fillings

Egg salad with chopped celery and olives; cream cheese with diced celery and green olives; cream cheese and peanut butter; cream cheese and raisins or chopped dates; mashed avocado with lemon juice and sprouts (ground almonds may be added, too); olive spread; peanut butter-celery spread; mushroom egg spread; carrot-apple-raisin sandwich filling; peanut butter carrot filling; grated cheddar cheese with mayonnaise, chopped green olives, chopped green onions, chopped pickle; baked beans and finely chopped onion on rye bread; peanut butter combined with apple or banana slices; cold buckwheat burgers on buns or stuffed in pita bread.

Blend equal parts of softened butter and cream cheese with a little mayonnaise and add any of the following: grated onion, chopped almonds, and a dash of curry powder; or grated cheddar and chopped parsley; or chopped pickle and green pepper.

Breads

Variety breads are a nice change for sandwiches. Try corn bread, rye bread, oatmeal bread, sprouted whole grain breads, whole wheat bagels, or pita bread.

Wide-Mouth Vacuum Bottle or Jar

Hot lentil, vegetable, potato or other soup; leftover heated casseroles; potato salad with egg; macaroni salad with cheese.

Extra-Added Attractions

Celery sticks with peanut butter, cream cheese and olive spread, or grated cheddar and chopped nuts; popcorn; sunflower seeds; dried fruit and nut combinations.

Desserts

Fresh fruit; dried fruit; natural cookies; carob brownies ....

And Don't Forget the Love!

Core an apple, pear, or other large fruit. Remove the core and slice the top third or so off. (Save the top. You'll need it again.) Write a little note or poem: "I love you! Have a wonderful day! I'm looking forward to seeing you this afternoon!" ... etc. Fold the note and wrap it in wax paper or foil, then slip it inside the cored fruit. Cover with the "lid." Stick toothpicks in to keep it stationary. Make a flag by attaching a piece of paper to a toothpick: "Look inside for a surprise!"

School Lunch Recipes

Cold Buckwheat Burgers

1 cup buckwheat (kasha)
2 cups water
1/2 teaspoon salt
1 tablespoon oil
1 clove garlic, slivered
1 medium onion, chopped
1 cup whole wheat flour
1/2 cup soy flour
1 tablespoon soy sauce

Bring salted water to boil and add buckwheat. Allow to boil for a moment, then reduce heat. Simmer, covered, for 15 to 20 minutes. Meanwhile, place frying pan on medium heat and add oil. Sauté garlic until well-browned. Add onion and stir for a few more minutes until lightly browned. Remove from heat. In a large mixing bowl, combine buckwheat, vegetables and flour. Mix thoroughly. When mixture has cooled enough to handle, form into balls 1 inch in diameter, then shape into patties. Return frying pan to medium-low heat and add just enough oil to coat bottom. Fry patties about 3 minutes on each side, turning often to assure even cooking. Add a sprinkle of soy sauce just before final turning. Makes about 12 burgers, which can be frozen until needed.

Mushroom-Egg Spread

3/4 cup finely diced mushrooms
3/4 cup finely diced onions
1/4 cup safflower oil
6 hard boiled eggs, mashed
1 teaspoon vegetable-flavored salt

Sauté mushrooms and onions. Cool. Combine with eggs, and add seasoning. Mix well!

Carrot-Apple-Raisin Filling

1 carrot, grated
1 apple, grated
1 tablespoon raisins
1 teaspoon chopped nuts
2 tablespoons mayonnaise

Combine all ingredients. Should make enough for 2 sandwiches.

Peanut Butter-Carrot Filling

3/4 cup peanut butter
2 tablespoons mayonnaise
1 1/2 cup finely grated carrot

Blend the above. Makes 2 1/2 cups. Add lettuce to sandwich.

Olive Spread

1 cup chopped ripe olives
1/2 cup finely chopped walnuts
1/4 cup finely chopped almonds
1/4 cup sunflower seeds (ground)
1/4 cup finely chopped celery

Combine with enough mayonnaise to moisten.

Peanut-Celery Spread

3 tablespoons peanut butter
2 tablespoons mayonnaise
4 tablespoons finely diced celery
2 tablespoons finely grated carrot
2 tablespoons chopped olives

Combine and salt to taste.

Appendix C

Suggested Reading List

This is a list of books that will help you in your explorations of the wonders and the health benefits of natural foods.

Children

Allergies and the Hyperactive Child, 2nd ed., Doris J. Rapp, edited by Madlyn Larsen. New York: Cornerstone Library, Inc., 1980.

Come and Get It—A Natural Foods Cookbook for Children, Kathleen M. Baxter. Ann Arbor, Mich.: Children First Press, 1981.

D C Super Heroes Super Healthy Cookbook—Good Food Kids Can Make Themselves, D C Comics. New York: Warner Books, Inc., 1981.

Earl Mindell's Vitamin Bible for Your Kids, Earl Mindell. New York: Rawson Wade Publishers, Inc., 1981.

Encyclopedia of Baby and Child Care, Lendon H. Smith. New York: Warner Books, Inc., 1980.

Feed Your Kids Right, Lendon Smith. New York: Dell Publishing Co., Inc., 1982.

Instant Baby Food, Linda McDonald. Pasadena, Calif.: Oaklawn Press, Inc., 1976.

Let's Have Healthy Children, rev. ed., Adelle Davis, revised by Marshall Mendel. New York: Signet Books, 1981.

Mommy, I'm Hungry: How to Feed Your Child Nutritiously, Patricia McEntire. Sacramento, Calif.: Cougar Books, 1982.

Nature's Children — A Guide to Organic Foods and Herbal Remedies for Children, Juliette De Bairacli-Levy. New York: Schocken Books, Inc., 1978.

Raising a Hyperactive Child, Mark A. Stewart and Sally W. Olds. New York: Harper and Row Publishers, Inc., 1973.

Consumer Information

Back to Eden, Jethro Kloss. Santa Barbara, Calif.: Woodbridge Press Publishing Co., 1981.

Complete Guide to Foot Reflexology, Kevin Kunz and Barbara Kunz. Englewood Cliffs, N.J.: Spectrum Books, 1980.

"Composition of Foods," Bernice K. Watt and Annabel L. Merrill, *Agriculture Handbook No. 8.* Agricultural Research Service, U.S. Department of Agriculture. Washington, D.C.: U.S. Government Printing Office.

Consumer Beware! Your Food and What's Been Done To It!, Beatrice T. Hunter. New York: Simon and Shuster, Inc., 1972.

Consumer's Dictionary of Cosmetic Ingredients, rev. ed., Ruth Winter. New York: Crown Publishing, Inc., 1976.

Consumer's Dictionary of Food Additives, Ruth Winter. New York: Crown Publishing, Inc., 1978.

Diet, Crime, and Delinquency, Alexander Schauss. Los Angeles, Calif.: Cancer Control Society.

Eater's Digest — The Consumer's Factbook of Food Additives, Michael F. Jacobson. Washington, D.C.: Center for Science in the Public Interest, 1982.

Physicians' Desk Reference for Nonprescription Drugs — 1981, Medical Economics Co. New York: Van Nostrand Reinhold Co., 1981.

Supermarket Handbook—Access to Whole Foods, Nikki Goldbeck and David Goldbeck. New York: Plume Books, 1974.

Your Healing Hands: The Polarity Experience, Richard Gordon. Santa Cruz, Calif.: Orenda Publishing/Unity Press, 1978.

Cookbooks

All Natural Soup Cookbook, Darcy Williamson and John Allgair, Bend, Oreg.: Maverick Publishing, 1982.

Beginner's Natural Food Cookbook, Judith Goeltz and Patricia Lazenby. Salt Lake City, Utah: Hawkes Publishing, Inc., 1975.

Good Breakfast Book: A Bringing-Back-Breakfast Cookbook, Nikki Goldbeck and David Goldbeck. New York: Quick Fox, 1976.

Let's Cook It Right, Adelle Davis. New York: Signet Books, 1970.

Natural Healing Cookbook: Over 450 Delicious Ways to Get Better and Stay Healthy, Mark Bricklin and Sharon Claessens. Emmaus, Penn.: Rodale Press Inc., 1981.

Rodale Cookbook, Nancy Albright. Emmaus, Penn.: Rodale Press Inc., 1973.

The 20-Minute Natural Foods Cookbook: Over 300 Kitchen-Tested Recipes, Sharon Claessens. Emmaus, Penn.: Rodale Press Inc., 1982.

Snacks

The Carob Way to Health, Frances S. Goulart. New York: Warner Books, 1982.

The Good Goodies—Recipes For Natural Snacks and Sweets, Stan Dworkin and Floss Dworkin. Emmaus, Penn.: Rodale Press Inc., 1974.

How To Survive Snack Attacks ... Naturally, Judi Zucker and Shari Zucker. Santa Barbara, Calif.: Woodbridge Press Publishing Co., 1979.

Natural Foods Sweet Tooth Cookbook, Eunice Farmilant. New York: Jove Publishing, Inc., 1978.

Snackers: Kick the Junk Food Habit, Maureen Wallace and Jim Wallace. Seattle, Wash.: Madrona Publishers, Inc., 1978.

Vegetarian

Book of Tofu, William Shurtleff and Akiko Aoyagi. New York: Ballantine Books, Inc., 1979.

Confessions of a Sneaky Organic Cook, Jean Kinderlehrer. New York: Signet Books.

Cooking What Comes Naturally — Vegetarian Recipes, rev. ed., Nikki Goldbeck. Woodstock, N.Y.: Ceres Press, 1981.

Deaf Smith Country Cookbook, J. F. Ford et al. New York: Collier, 1973.

Fresh Vegetable and Fruit Juices, rev. ed., N. W. Walker. Phoenix, Ariz.: Norwalk Press, 1970.

Great Meatless Meals, Frances M. Lappe and Ellen B. Ewald. New York: Ballantine, 1981.

Here's To You, Honey: The Book That Takes Up Where the World of Honey Leaves Off, vol. 2, Joe M. Parkhill, Berryville, Ark.: Country Bazaar Publishing, 1980.

How To Eat Without Meat ... Naturally, Judi Zucker and Shari Zucker. Santa Barbara, Calif.: Woodbridge Press Publishing Co., 1981.

Kathy Cooks ... Naturally, Kathy Hoshijo. San Francisco: Harbor Publishing, Inc., 1981.

Laurel's Kitchen: A Handbook for Vegetarian Cookery and Nutrition, Laurel Robertson et al. New York: Bantam Books, Inc., 1978.

Recipes for a Small Planet, Ellen B. Ewald. New York: Ballantine Books, Inc., 1975.

Recipes for Longer Life, Ann Wigmore. Edited by Betsy Kimball. Boston, Mass.: Hippocrates Press.

Simpler Life Cookbook: From Arrowhead Mills, Frank Ford. Waco, Tex.: Harvest Press, Inc., 1978.

Sprout For the Love of Everybody: Nutritional Evaluation of Sprouts and Grasses, Viktoras Kulvinskas. Fairfield, Iowa: Twenty First Century Publishing.

Ten Talents Cookbook: Vegetarian Natural Foods, Frank J. Hurd and Rosalie Hurd. Chisholm, Minn.: Ten Talents, 1968.

The Uncook Book — Raw Food Adventures to a New Health High, Elizabeth Baker and Elton Baker. Portland, Oreg.: Drelwood Publishing, 1981.

Vital Foods — Total Health, Bernard D. Jensen. Los Angeles, Calif.: Cancer Control Society.

Disease

Allergies and Your Family, Doris J. Rapp. New York: Sterling Publishing Co., Inc. 1980.

Cancer — A Total Approach, Paavo Airola. Phoenix, Ariz.: Health Plus Publishing.

Cancer Therapy: Fifty Cases, Max Gerson. Los Angeles, Calif.: Cancer Control Society.

The Death of Cancer, Harold Manner. Los Angeles, Calif.: Cancer Control Society.

Do It Yourself Allergy Analysis Handbook, Kate Ludeman and Louise Henderson. New Canaan, Conn.: Keats Publishing, Inc., 1979.

Dr. Mandell's Allergy-Free Cookbook, Marshall Mandell and Fran Gare. New York: Pocket Books, Inc., 1981.

Hypoglycemia: A Better Approach, Paavo Airola. Phoenix, Ariz.: Health Plus Publishing, 1977.

One Answer to Cancer, William Kelley. Los Angeles, Calif.: Cancer Control Society.

Tracking Down Hidden Food Allergy, 2nd ed., William G. Crook. Jackson, Tenn.: Professional Books, 1980.

Macrobiotics

Calendar Cookbook, Cornelia Aihara. Oroville, Calif.: George Ohsawa, Macrobiotics Foundation, 1979.

Healing Miracles From Macrobiotics, Kohler. Englewood Cliffs, N.J.: Prentice-Hall, Inc., 1982.

Macrobiotic Cooking For Everyone, Edward Esko and Wendy Esko. Scranton, Penn.: Japan Publishing, Inc., 1980.

Natural Healing Through Macrobiotics, Michio Kushi. Scranton, Penn.: Japan Publishing, Inc., 1979.

You Are All Sanpaku, George Ohsawa. Secaucus, N.J.: University Books, Inc., 1980

Zen Macrobiotic Cooking, Michel Abehsera. New York: Avon Books, 1970.

Nutrition

Anatomy of an Illness, As Perceived by the Patient, Norman Cousins. New York: Bantam Books, Inc., 1981.

Are You Confused? Paavo Airola. Forward by Leslie H. Salov. Phoenix, Ariz.: Health Plus Publishing, 1971.

Beverly Hills Medical Diet, Arnold Fox. New York: Bantam Books, Inc., 1982.

Complete Book of Minerals for Health, rev. ed. Emmaus, Penn.: Rodale Press, Inc., 1981.

Complete Handbook of Nutrition, Gary Null and Steve Null, Health Library, vol. 1. New York: Dell Publishing Co., Inc., 1972.

Diet and Nutrition – Holistic Approach, R. M. Ballentine. Honesdale, Penn.: Himalayan International Institute, 1978.

Discovering Natural Foods, Roy Bruder. Santa Barbara, Calif.: Woodbridge Press Publishing Co., 1982.

Dr. Atkins' Nutrition Breakthrough: How to Treat Your Medical Condition Without Drugs, Robert C. Atkins. New York: Bantam Books Inc., 1982.

Food Combining Handbook, Gary Null et al. New York: Jove Publications, Inc., 1973.

Food Is Your Best Medicine, Henry Bieler. New York: Ballantine Books Inc., 1982.

Health Secrets From Europe, Paavo O. Airola, New York: Arco Publishing, Inc., 1971.

Herb Book, edited by John Lust. New York: Bantam Books, Inc., 1974.

Herbs and Things—Jeanne Rose's Herbal, Jeanne Rose. New York: Grosset and Dunlap, Inc., 1972.

How To Get Well: Dr. Airola's Handbook of Natural Healing, Paavo Airola. Phoenix, Ariz.: Health Plus Publishing, 1974.

The Kamen Plan for Total Nutrition During Pregnancy, Betty Kamen and Si Kamen. East Norwalk, Conn.: Appleton-Century-Crofts, 1981.

Killer Salt, new ed., Marietta Whittlesey. New York: Bolder Books, Inc., 1977.

Let's Eat Right To Keep Fit, Adelle Davis. New York: Signet Books, 1970.

Maximum Life Span, Roy L. Walford. New York: W. W. Norton & Co., 1983.

Miracle of Fasting, 30th ed., Paul C. Bragg and Patricia Bragg. Santa Barbara: Health Science.

Nutrition Almanac, rev. ed., edited by John D. Kirschmann. New York: McGraw-Hill Book Co., 1979.

The People's Guide to Vitamins and Minerals: From A to Zinc, Dominick Bosco. Chicago, Ill.: Contemporary Books, Inc., 1980.

Nutrition and Your Mind, George Watson. New York: Bantam Books, Inc., 1974.

Sugar Blues, William Dufty. New York: Warner Books, Inc., 1976.

Supernutrition for Healthy Hearts, Richard Passwater. New York: Jove Publishing, Inc., 1978.

Survival into the Twenty-First Century, Viktoras Kulvinskas. Edited by Hermine Hurlbut and Joan Newman. Fairfield, Iowa: Twenty First Century Publishing, 1975.

Vitamins and You, Robert J. Benowicz. New York: Berkeley Publishing Corp., 1981.

Way of Herbs—Simple Remedies for Health and Healing, Michael Tierra. Santa Cruz, Calif.: Orenda Publishing/Unity Press, 1980.

We Love Your Body, Lani Miller and Diane Rodgers. Seattle, Wash.: Morse Press, Inc., 1980.

Women

Childbirth Without Fear, rev., 4th ed., Grantley Dick-Reade. New York: Harper and Row Publishing Inc., 1978.

Everywoman's Book, Paavo Airola. Phoenix, Ariz.: Health Plus Publishing, 1979.